Case Studies in Non-directive Play Therapy

Yet for this we travelled
With hope, and not alone,
In the country of ourselves
                    Theodore Roethke, 'The Harsh Country'

Case Studies in Non-directive Play Therapy

Virginia Ryan
BA *summa cum laude*, PhD, CPsychol
Honorary Fellow
Department of Social Policy and Professional Studies
University of Hull
Co-facilitator, Post-qualifying Training
Programme in Non-directive Play Therapy,
Department of Social Policy and Social Work
University of York

Kate Wilson
BA(Oxon), DipSW, Dip Couns
Senior Lecturer in Social Work
Director, Post-qualifying Training
Department of Social Policy and Social Work
University of York
York, UK

Baillière Tindall
London   Philadelphia   Toronto   Sydney   Tokyo

Baillière Tindall   24–28 Oval Road
                      London NW1 7DX

                      The Curtis Center
                      Independence Square West
                      Philadelphia, PA 19106–3399, USA

                      Harcourt Brace & Company
                      55 Horner Avenue
                      Toronto, Ontario, M8Z 4X6, Canada

                      Harcourt Brace & Company, Australia
                      30–52 Smidmore Street
                      Marrickville
                      NSW 2204, Australia

                      Harcourt Brace & Company, Japan
                      Ichibancho Central Building
                      22–1 Ichibancho
                      Chiyoda-ku, Tokyo 102, Japan

© 1996 Baillière Tindall

This book is printed on acid-free paper

All rights reserved. No part of this publication may be reproduced, stored in a retrieval system or transmitted, in any form or by any other means, electronic, mechanical, photocopying or otherwise, without the prior permission of Baillère Tindall, 24–28 Oval Road, London NW1 7DX

A catalogue record for this book is available from the British Library

ISBN 0-7020-1830-9

Typeset by J&L Composition Ltd, Filey, North Yorkshire
Printed and bound in Great Britain by WBC Book Manufacturers, Bridgend, Glamorgan

Contents

Acknowledgements	vii

Introduction: Non-directive Play Therapy with
Emotionally Damaged Children ... 1

Chapter 1
Susan: Beginning Play Therapy ... 11
Theoretical Issue: The underlying assumptions of non-directive play therapy ... 21
Practice Issues: Working therapeutically with children in statutory settings ... 25
Introductory meetings ... 33

Chapter 2
Patrick: From Concrete to Symbolic Play ... 40
Practice Issues: Communicating with young children ... 54
Responding to allegations of abuse made during therapy ... 58
Using other therapeutic skills and the therapeutic value of routines ... 62
Theoretical Issue: Restoring a child's normal developmental trajectory within play therapy ... 64

Chapter 3
Diane: Repairing and Creating Identity ... 71
Practice Issues: Role-playing within non-directive play therapy
Evaluating therapeutic progress ... 87
Theoretical Issue: Physical abuse and non-directive play therapy ... 94

Chapter 4
Anna: A Silent Communication ... 102
Practice Issues: Working with silence ... 117
Reworking traumatic memories in therapy ... 123
Ending therapy ... 125
Theoretical Issues: Children's responses to divorce ... 127
Individual help or family conciliation ... 131
Contact with the non-custodial parent ... 132

Chapter 5
Delroy: A Child Without Support 135
Theoretical Issues: Attachment issues within a play therapy
context 149
Emotional and intellectual impairment and
its links with epilepsy 152
Practice Issues: Race, gender and power within play therapy 155
Personal issues for the therapist 157

Chapter 6
Patricia: Reworking Abusive Experiences in Adolescence 159
Practice Issues: Adapting play therapy to the needs of
adolescents 172
Theoretical Issues: The development of adult identity 178
The reworking of sexually abusive experiences
in play therapy 183

Chapter 7
Ben: A Therapeutic Assessment for the Court 188
Practice Issues: Differences and similarities between
assessments and sustained therapeutic work 206
Restrictions on conducting therapeutic
assessments 216
Other methods of psychological assessment 219
Confidentiality and recording in court
assessments 221
Working with other professionals 224
Theoretical Issue: Distinguishing the child's wishes, feelings and
fantasies from real current and past life events 226

References 234
Index 241

Acknowledgments

Once again we thank our families for their support and sustenance while we wrote this book. Kate's mother, Anne Ridler, in particular attempted to help us with our rough-and-ready narrative style and our literary sources, but is not responsible for our shortcomings! We are also very grateful to colleagues who consented to read and comment on chapters in preparation: Paula Kendrick, whom we sorely missed after our ideal partnership in our first book, but who understandably was too busy practicing this time around; Celia Downes, for reading 'Patricia'; Adrian James, for his useful comments on 'Anna'; Dorothy Heard and Brian Lake for their theoretical expertise; Alison Holdsworth, for helping us at short notice with the typing; and Anna Markowycz, for reading 'Ben' from a guardian's viewpoint. Virginia also wishes to thank Dr. Roger Williams for looking at part of 'Ben', and more generally for his consultations/supervisions. These have been invaluable to her personal and professional development, particularly in the area of therapeutic assessments. We wish to thank Charlotte McSherry and all the other children at St Vincent's R.C. School, Hull for their help with our cover.

Introduction
Non-directive Play Therapy with Emotionally Damaged Children

This book, which is intended as a companion to our earlier book on play therapy, is based on a number of case examples of play therapy with children and adolescents, derived from the practice of one of the authors, Virginia Ryan. Our purpose in writing the book is, through the detailed accounts of sessions with these individual children and the supporting discussion of them, to provide guidance on the practice skills and techniques of non-directive play therapy, and the attitudes and thinking which lie behind the method. We intend the book to be used by experienced practitioners and students, but hope that it will also be useful as an introduction for a parent or carer whose child has been offered non-directive play therapy and for readers with a general interest in the subject.

In this introduction, before explaining in more detail how we have designed the book, we provide a brief overview and introduction to non-directive play therapy as an approach. Since our earlier book discusses this more fully, we shall here only give an outline of its main characteristics, its historical origins and its theoretical underpinnings, but in sufficient detail, we hope, to enable this book to stand on its own and to provide a framework for the chapters which follow. Although many topics relating to both theory and practice are considered in the individual chapters, the interested reader will need to refer to the earlier book for a fuller account of, say, planning and preparation for play therapy, or of symbolic play and its role in mental development and play therapy.

The method used with all the children whose therapy is described in the book is that of non-directive play therapy. This approach is based on Rogerian client-centred therapy with adults (Rogers, 1976), adapted to child therapy, and uses play rather than verbal exchange as the principal means of communication. It differs from other play interventions and therapies primarily in its 'non-directive' stance: that is, the choice of issues and activity in the playroom is determined by the child rather than the adult, within certain basic limits set by the therapist. A relationship is built up between child and therapist, in which the child with the therapist's help, develops the freedom to choose the feelings he or she wishes to explore, and the means through which to do this. These feelings may be communicated both directly and indirectly through the child's actions, language and play. The therapist's role is to listen, understand and respond to the child, thus facilitating the latter's awareness of thoughts and feelings, particularly those which are conflicting and confused. This reflection process is akin to Stern's concept of infant/carer attunement (Stern, 1985), but is employed in a heightened, more self-conscious and self-controlled manner by the therapist in comparison to a carer. Unlike some other therapeutic methods with children, this reflection process by the therapist does not include praising, interpretation of underlying motivation, problem-solving or undermining the child's defences. The non-directive method assumes that the child will instigate therapeutic changes and achieve therapeutic insights with the therapist's support, but without her overt directions. The child can then freely use the playroom and the therapist to resolve emotional difficulties at his or her own pace, and to achieve emotional relaxation and self-control.

The therapist's role and task, then, within the approach is characterised by a number of features, of which the following are the most important.

1. The creation of a permissive, child-centred atmosphere. This is in part developed because the child is allowed to choose the focus of activity within the therapy sessions and in part because the therapist's friendly, attentive, consistent but non-intrusive attitude gradually enables the child to feel secure in her presence.
2. The setting of therapeutic limits to the child's behaviour, in order to ensure the child's safety and security within the playroom.
3. The recognition of what the child is experiencing, and the reflection of this understanding to the child in a non-threatening manner. The therapist's generalised attitude of attentiveness and understanding is communicated through 'emotive messages' in which the feelings, thoughts and wishes she has about the child's behaviour are expressed both verbally and through non-verbal means, including voice tone, gesture and facial expression (Heard and Lake, 1986).

The underlying philosophy of the approach has traditionally followed the Rogerian theory of normal personality development and conflict resolution, namely that there exists in all human beings a drive for self-realisation, i.e. a drive towards maturity, independence and uniqueness. It assumes that individuals at any age have within themselves not only the ability to solve their problems satisfactorily, but also a striving for growth which makes mature behaviour more satisfying than immature behaviour, given minimally satisfying conditions.

The method was developed primarily by Virginia Axline, in two books first published in the 1940s, which have continued to be read widely by professional audiences in North America, the UK and to a lesser extent in other northern European countries. The first of these, *Dibs: In Search of Self* (1946), consists of an extended case-study of play therapy with a six year old boy; the second (1947) sets out eight principles of practice which are linked to a discussion of the therapeutic process through numerous practice examples. Other major contributors to the development of the approach have been Moustakas (1953) and Ginott (1961). Non-directive play therapy, as it became known in Britain, seems to have been practised in relative isolation at child guidance and treatment centres, and there have been other, separate developments in continental Europe, notably in Germany and Holland (van der Kooij and Hellendorn, 1986).

However, for reasons discussed elsewhere (Ryan, 1995a), the method has failed to develop into a major school of therapy in the way that other therapies have done. The techniques involved have often not been clearly specified or linked to theoretical principles, and there has been a tendency to drift into other therapeutic techniques. More recently, and this is probably true of other therapeutic approaches as well, the need to consider practice issues which arise from its use in statutory child care has become evident. The foundations of therapeutic approaches to working with children were largely established before state intervention came to play such a central part in child welfare. Many of the issues, therefore, which we consider in this book (for example the need for an adequately supportive environment, contacts between carers, social workers and therapist, the limits to confidentiality, and the relationship between therapeutic work and work for the courts, to name but a few) now have to be reconsidered in relation both to the principles of the non-directive approach and to the current child welfare context in which it is practised.

A number of recent books and book chapters have begun to review and update the practice of non-directive play therapy; its procedures and theoretical foundations have begun to be more rigorously specified (see, for example, Guerney, 1984; West, 1992; Wilson et al., 1992). We hope that this present book will provide a useful addition to this growing body of literature. However, there still remains a need for more tightly specified theoretical links to current developments in attachment theory and research. Process and outcome research is also required in order to assess both the longer-term effectiveness of the method and also the effectiveness of its techniques in a child welfare context.

THE THEORETICAL BASIS OF NON-DIRECTIVE PLAY THERAPY

Non-directive play therapy has been given a firm foundation in current child development principles in our first book and was set, following Piaget, within a broad developmental framework of adaptation. In this framework, all of a child's activities are assumed to further adaptation to his or her environment; the developing child gradually moves from simple built-in sensori-motor schemas to the more internalised, increasingly complex mental categories seen in later childhood. Adaptation is said to occur by means of two basic processes: assimilation and accommodation. The active internalisation of experiences by a child, or assimilation, is the process whereby children seek to incorporate new experiences into their existing repertoire of schemas and is a child's most basic and elementary activity. The complementary process to this is accommodation. This is the child's other main adaptive function; it involves the alteration of internal schemas and the adjustment of the child's activity to take account of new information about the environment.

These mental schemas are made up of affective, cognitive and motor components. Personal schemas (primarily those involving relationships) are mainly affective, but it is assumed that affect, cognition and motor responses are involved in each mental state, although the degree of each component varies. While conceptually separate, these components are experientially inseparable for the child.

In normal development, unlike the development of emotionally damaged children, the large majority of the child's personally significant experiences are positive ones (Erikson, 1963). These experiences will result in relatively permanent mental schemas on all three cognitive, motor and emotional levels of functioning, and will be based not only on the child's relationships with carers but will also crucially incorporate fundamental aspects of the child's ideas about the self (these correspond to attachment theorists' 'multiple models of the self'). Negative experiences, although present, are not as emotionally salient nor nearly as frequent as positive ones, and indeed, as Dunn (1988) implies, within an overall benign context of family relationships, may in fact help the child in achieving strong and flexible personal schemas.

In normal mental development, then, the child will have developed (and will be in the process of further developing) relatively permanent schemas towards his or her carers, for example, schemas of trust, love and dependency. These schemas will incorporate the child's strong positive feelings towards the carers, as well as weaker and less powerful negative affect, for example, jealousy, resentment and anger. 'Personal schemas' correspond to the internal mental representations posited by attachment theorists which are assumed to develop in primary attachment relationships (Bretherton and Waters, 1985).

With emotionally damaged children, however, the affective, motor and cognitive components of their personal schemas are assumed to be more distorted, conflicting and/or dissociated from one another than normal because of the more strongly negative experiences they have had with their carers, alongside their positive experiences (see also Main and Hesse, 1990). Repeated abusive experiences, or even a single traumatic event, may lead a child to develop strongly negative or conflicting personal schemas about the self and significant others. The need to protect the self against the potentially damaging or unpredictable behaviour of carers may lead to the development of overly accommodating responses such as passivity, or regression to less mature levels of functioning, which frequently characterise the behaviour of damaged children.

Using this framework, then, emotionally damaged children may be viewed as having been subjected to experiences in which they have had to over-accommodate to the environment, rather than freely assimilating their experiences to personal schemas as the child abuse and neglect research literature implies. As a result, these children's personal schemas will not be as easily assimilated to one another and even a highly compensatory environment, such as that for example provided by loving and responsive foster carers, may be insufficient to enable a child to abandon these previously adaptive mental schemas for more positive ones. The child may need an intensive, corrective experience such as that provided in non-directive play therapy in order to re-enact emotionally damaging experiences on a symbolic level and to effect a re-alignment of personal schemas.

One universal and highly assimilative activity for a child is symbolic play. A child who is engaged in symbolic play, either under everyday conditions or during non-directive play therapy, spontaneously assimilates personally meaningful experiences to internal, mental structures, or schemas. During symbolic play, a child can largely ignore external environmental constraints on mental activity, at the same time as he freely assimilates personal experiences. (For example, a child astride a broom handle can ignore what it actually is as he pretends to be a rider on a horse.)

In contrast to the non-abused child, a troubled or abused child may not be able readily to use an assimilating device such as symbolic play. However, in a permissive, enhanced play environment, such as that provided in non-directive play therapy, the child is offered the opportunity of using a symbolic means, namely play, to work through conflicts which may exist at an affective, cognitive and motor level. The non-threatening, therapeutic environment enables him or her during symbolic play to assimilate personal experiences freely. Coupled with the therapist's focus on the child's feelings and the setting of certain limits to behaviour, the following changes are assumed to occur.

1. Thoughts and feelings previously outside the child's awareness are made conscious and given symbolic representation.
2. Because of the child's increased symbolic assimilation during therapy, the internal organisation of schemas changes and connections with other personal schemas also alter.
3. Schemas become more mobile in assimilating new events to past experiences, resulting in changes of the child's mental organisation and structure (i.e. personality change) and changes in the child's behaviour.

This, then, is the theoretical framework in which we set non-directive play therapy, and within which the detailed work with the individual children recounted in the following chapters needs to be understood. Some of the discussion in individual chapters provides a more detailed illustration of these theoretical foundations, which will, because they are related to specific examples, we hope be more readily understood in this context. We now explain the way in which we have organised the book.

AN OVERVIEW OF OUR APPROACH IN THIS BOOK

We have chosen our examples from a range of the children with whom Virginia Ryan has worked during the past several years, in order to provide a detailed illustration of the process of play therapy, and a discussion of the theoretical and practice issues raised by each account. We are conscious that books on play therapy rarely address, through sustained description of work with individual children, the underlying issues involved in therapeutic interventions. We hope, through the approach adopted here, that we shall illustrate not only the practice skills and techniques but also some of the theoretical and practice considerations which need to be considered in this method of therapeutic work. In selecting our particular examples (some of which, as we explain below, are composite ones) we have tried to choose children from a range of circumstances, family background, age and gender, and whose therapy sessions seemed best to illustrate the dimensions of play therapy which we consider to be of critical importance.

Each chapter, broadly speaking, is divided into three parts: the first section provides a clinical example, with a brief background to the child followed by an account of the play therapy sessions undertaken with him or her; the second section explores one or more of the theoretical topics; and the third section considers some of the practice issues raised by this therapeutic intervention. We have varied the format of the individual chapters slightly and also adapted the way in which we present the clinical material to the particular topics which we have chosen to consider.

Inevitably, because the majority of Virginia's work is with children who have been referred for play therapy by local authorities, most of those whom we have described here have had abusive experiences (and indeed, the one child, Anna, who was seen privately, had certainly been a witness to violent episodes between her parents). However, in the discussions which follow each account, we have tried not to repeat points which, although relevant to work with a particular child, are explored elsewhere in the book in relation to a different case. We do not always consider, say, how an abusive experience emerged and was responded to, even though this may well have been an important theme in the play therapy. For example, some of the behaviours which Delroy showed in his sessions strongly supported earlier allegations that he had been sexually abused. Although we illustrate in this clinical account the way in which the therapist should respond to sexualised behaviours, we do not explore this issue or the issue of disclosure during therapy sessions in this chapter since they are considered in other chapters (Patrick and Patricia).

A particularly difficult issue for us in writing the book has been to protect the privacy of the individual children about whom we are writing. This is especially so, since, unlike adults, children are not able to give informed consent for their therapeutic material to be put into print. It did not always seem possible to preserve the integrity of each child's unique experience and at the same time respect the child's right to anonymity. As a result, in order to ensure confidentiality, we have in some cases, in addition to altering identifying background information and details of the content of the sessions, combined two or more children's material into composite examples. In these cases, the children all had strong psychological similarities in the particular areas described, even though other aspects of their life story and play therapy sessions were not the same.

We realise that it is a natural instinct, when reading about an individual, to want to know what happened next. Quite apart from a professional concern about the effectiveness of the intervention, it reflects a deep-seated urge in most of us to know 'the end of the story'. Where we have been in a position to do so, we have given a brief indication of the outcome for the child on whom the study is primarily based. Detailed outcomes, however, are not appropriate, not least because this has not been the focus or approach of the book. We hope to address these issues more thoroughly through collected and analysed results in planned process and outcome research.

We begin our book with a chapter in which we explore issues in planning and beginning therapy, discussing the initial stages of work with a six year old in foster care. We describe the introductory meetings with Susan and her brothers, with her birth parents and with her foster carers, and then give a detailed account of Susan's first play therapy session. There follows a discussion of the underlying theoretical assumptions of non-directive play therapy, the way in which the therapist's responses in the first session reflected the core features of the approach, and how Susan's therapeutic progress became evident in her later sessions. The section on practice issues discusses some of the practice considerations at referral, including: the need to consider the appropriateness of individual therapy and the supportiveness of the child's environment; working with foster carers; issues which may arise in introductory meetings; and the internal mental focus which the therapist needs to attain during her first session with the child.

In Chapter 2, we give an account of the play therapy sessions undertaken with a four year old, Patrick, who had been sexually and emotionally abused before being removed from the care of his parents and placed in a foster home. The sessions illustrate the ways in which a child can move from very concrete, circumscribed play to develop the more normal capacity to play on a symbolic level. The discussion which follows considers some of the practice issues involved in working with a child with rudimentary language development, as well as the role of the therapist when allegations of abuse are made by the child during play therapy sessions. In the section on theoretical issues, we examine the notion of play therapy as an artificially enhanced environment, the links between an understanding of normal development and the assessment of a child's therapeutic progress, and the role of symbolisation in play therapy and normal development.

In our next chapter, we describe the fifteen play therapy sessions undertaken with a ten year old girl, Diane. During her therapy, Diane's personality changed from being passive and rather listless to that of a lively and in many respects outgoing child, and her therapy sessions show the imaginative and creative ways through which she chose to address her earlier damaging experiences. In the section on practice issues which follows, we consider the therapist's role within role plays devised by the child, and ways of evaluating therapeutic progress. The final theoretical section considers physical abuse and its impact on a child within a framework of mental development, and how its effects emerged as themes in Diane's play.

We have called our next chapter, which describes play therapy with a seven year old girl whose parents were in the throes of divorce, 'a silent communication', since during her initial ten sessions Anna was almost entirely silent. In our discussion of practice issues, we consider first ways of understanding and working in silence, second the reworking of earlier traumatic experiences in therapy and third, decisions about the appropriate time to end therapy. In our final section, we consider the impact of parental separation on children and link this with what emerged in Anna's therapy; and finally we consider the appropriateness of individual work as opposed to family conciliation.

Chapter 5 describes twelve play therapy sessions undertaken with an eight year old, mixed-race boy, who suffered from epilepsy. Although some therapeutic progress is evident in his sessions, the outcome for Delroy was not successful, and in our discussion of theoretical issues, we consider some of the reasons for this, focusing in particular on the significance of attachment relationships and the way in which the dearth of even temporary attachments rendered therapeutic intervention ineffective. The inter-relationship between emotional and physical factors, in this case, Delroy's emotional neglect, sexual abuse and epilepsy, are explored. In our final section on practice issues, which in this chapter for reasons of clarity we put after that on theoretical topics, we consider issues of race, gender and power in therapy, and personal issues for the therapist which came to the fore in working with Delroy but have, we think, general relevance.

We wanted to show that a play therapy approach, if appropriately modified, can also be successful in addressing the needs of older children and adolescents. Our next chapter, therefore, describes play therapy with a thirteen year old girl, who was in care as a result of alleging that her uncle and later her step-father had sexually abused her. We discuss Patricia's fifteen sessions through the themes which emerged in them, namely confidentiality and trusting adults, the reworking of sexually abusive experiences on a motor level, and relationships with peers and other significant adults. In our discussion of practice issues, we consider the way in which play therapy needs to be adapted to working with adolescents. In the concluding section on theoretical topics, we consider the development of an adult sense of identity during adolescence, and how Patricia's therapy illustrated this process. Finally, we discuss our theoretical understanding of the impact which sexual abuse has on the individual's sense of self, and the way in which non-directive play therapy addresses this impact.

Our concluding chapter considers non-directive play therapy as a method of assessment which may be used in court proceedings. We explore this through an account of five sessions which were undertaken with Ben, a nine year old boy, in order to help him express his needs, wishes and feelings through play sessions, and to enable the therapist to give an opinion on his future needs to the court. Although this kind of intervention is essentially conducted in the same manner as the longer-term work described in our earlier chapters, it raises particular issues, which we consider in the practice and theoretical sections. In the former section, assessment issues, and issues such as those of confidentiality, therapeutic suggestion, and the writing of court reports based on play sessions are explored. In the latter section, we discuss ways in which the therapist distinguishes between material which expresses a child's wishes, feelings and fantasies, and that which reflects actual current or past events in the child's life.

Finally, a word about the stylistic conventions of the book. The accounts of the play therapy itself in each chapter are written in the first person, since they describe, as we have said, work undertaken by one of the authors. The practice and theory sections are written in the third person, reflecting the combined ideas of both authors. In these, we have adopted the convention of calling the practitioner 'therapist', since this seemed the most appropriate terminology. As always, we have struggled with the gender of the third person singular. We have generally adopted, for the child, the masculine form, to distinguish this from the therapist, whom we have, since both the authors are women, referred to as 'she'.

We are very much aware that these case studies give only a partial and incomplete account of non-directive play therapy, and that many issues raised by them remain unexplored. We hope nonetheless to demonstrate in the book our belief that individual child therapy has an important part to play in current treatment plans for families. Although discussion of different kinds of treatment is outside the scope of this book, we consider that play therapy certainly does not preclude seeing families and siblings together, supporting and counselling children's carers, or conducting groupwork for children, all of which can be appropriate at certain times in an individual's life, and for certain families (as we argue elsewhere: Wilson and Ryan, 1994a). Equally, we hope these case studies will demonstrate that non-directive play therapy can be an effective and relatively short-term means of providing children with the time, space and intensive adult help necessary for self-learning and self-growth.

Chapter 1

Susan
Beginning Play Therapy

*Like dust in a whirlwind, making
The wild wind visible*

Robinson Jeffers

In this chapter we explore issues in planning and beginning play therapy by discussing the initial stages of work with Susan, a six-year-old child who, together with her two brothers, was in local authority care. In our earlier book (Wilson et al., 1992, chapter 3) we considered general issues and planning tasks in beginning play therapy. However, because practice issues are often more complicated in statutory work, particularly because of the need to work with birth parents, foster carers and other professionals, we now consider these early stages explicitly. We begin with an account of Susan's background, introductory meetings and her first session, which we describe in detail. There follows a discussion of the underlying theoretical assumptions of non-directive play therapy, the way the core features of the approach guided the therapist in this first session and Susan's therapeutic progress on her evolving concerns. The final section considers some of the practice issues involved in the preparatory stages of therapy.

SUSAN'S BACKGROUND

Susan was referred to me for play therapy by her social worker together with her older brother, Gerry, aged eight, and her younger brother, Mark, aged four. Although Susan's progress in therapy was influenced significantly by the individual play therapy sessions undertaken simultaneously with her brothers, the children's referral and their play therapy sessions will be considered only from Susan's perspective.

At our referral meeting both the social worker, John, and the children's foster carer, Cath, were present. The immediate reason for referral was that the children seemed extremely upset by visits with their natural parents. These visits caused the children to become greatly agitated: Susan became even more anxious than usual to please everyone; Gerry and Mark became more aggressive with one another; and Susan and Mark often had night-time enuresis both before and after the visits. The children's behaviour during contacts alternated between very passive, withdrawn behaviour and aggressive play with one another, with little positive interaction between the children and their parents. John's and his team leader's efforts to direct both the parents' and children's attention to better communication with one another had been unsuccessful.

John had applied to the court temporarily to suspend these visits, an action supported by the children's foster carers, Cath and her husband, Edward, with whom the children had been staying since being separated from their parents. The children had been on the local authority's child protection register for children at risk of significant harm under the category 'neglect' since Mark's birth. The parents' care of the three children had been poor, even with extensive support and guidance. Eight months ago the health visitor had seen severe bruising on Mark's head and face during one of her routine visits; a physical examination at the hospital concluded that the injuries were consistent with Mark having been beaten and injured deliberately by two adults, one of them more physically powerful than the other. Care Orders on all the children were granted at the final hearing three months ago, where a finding of fact was made by the judge that Mark had been physically injured by his parents and all the children had been neglected. Monthly contact visits between the children and their parents were also agreed in accordance with the local authority care plan, which was for the children to remain together in their current placement on a long-term basis.

Susan herself was described to me as small in stature, rather thin, with blond hair and light brown eyes. Both John and Cath were concerned that, although Susan had made some progress in their care, she was still overly compliant and easily upset, even without parental visits. She dissolved into tears frequently and automatically followed what her brothers, peers or any adults told her to do, regardless of her own feelings. A recent educational assessment of Susan described her as lagging approximately two years behind her chronological age academically. This developmental delay, the educational psychologist wrote, was most probably due to a combination of factors: Susan's test results showed a low general intellectual ability; emotional factors, in particular her passivity and overcompliance, also seemed to hinder her progress. In addition, Susan was said to exhibit a low impulse control and poor concentration.

At our meeting we also discussed the implications for Cath and Edward of the children attending play therapy. While I stressed that the pace of therapy was the child's own choice, I also stated that sometimes a child did begin to unearth difficult thoughts and emotions during sessions, as well as new ways of responding to situations and people. These could carry over to everyday events. Of course, I added, this was the goal of therapy sessions, to influence the child to change. However, sometimes a child responded with negative behaviour, such as tantrums, sleep disturbance or tenseness for a short time before relaxing and settling into new-found ways of responding to people. Carers needed to be more flexible and more supportive in their responses in order to adapt to any changes in the child.

It was agreed that we would all meet once a month for progress meetings, where I would give an indication of the children's general therapeutic progress and we could discuss the children's behaviour at home. The foster carers would also have regular weekly meetings with John, in addition to the support from their foster leader. I would arrange to meet the children's parents to explain my role to them.

The last part of our referral meeting was spent discussing the practicalities of time, place and transport. Cath and I arranged that I would introduce myself to the children at home a short while before I began my play therapy sessions with them. Finally, John gave me access to Susan's and her brothers' files to supplement any information I had been given orally. I arranged for court reports, other professionals' reports and contact notes to be sent to me and read some of the most pertinent ones before I met the children myself. I also agreed to write a report for the court on all three children's needs, wishes and feelings regarding contact with their parents, based on their play therapy sessions with me.

INTRODUCTORY VISITS

Meeting the children

My meeting with Susan and her brothers took place in the playroom at their foster home. After Cath introduced them to me, Gerry continued to play on his hand-held computer game and Susan rushed around the room with a doll's pram. Mark sat very close to me on the couch and talked rapidly to me about his morning's activities, trying to have my exclusive attention. When Mark paused I said that maybe Cath had told them that their social worker, John, had asked me to see them in my playroom. My job was to try to help children who were worried and unhappy or afraid of things. I had already talked with John and Cath: 'They said that maybe I can help you'.

None of the children looked at me or responded when I paused, but their unnatural stillness was an indication to me that they were listening intently:

V: [gently] Maybe you don't know what to think about what I said. [Pause]

V: [continuing] When you come to see me, you can play with things or talk, or just sit with me. You'll each have a turn by yourself in the playroom. It will be time for you to choose what you want to do there. [Pause]

V: Cath will wait for you in another room and you can be with her when you're waiting for your turn. . . . Maybe I can tell you about my playroom. It's in a building near the park. I can draw the building for you now and then you'd know what it looks like.

As I found a piece of paper and a pen in my bag, Susan and Gerry moved closer to Mark, and Mark said he wanted to draw. I got more paper and pens out of my bag, and talked about the building and the park. As Mark and I drew, Susan and Gerry watched closely and listened to me as I described the playroom and what was in it. I then talked about when they would come to see me and how many times and for how long. I also said that sometimes other children might ask Gerry, and maybe Susan and Mark where they went on Wednesdays. Everybody could say that they were going to a playroom for some special time or maybe Gerry or Cath had an idea of what to say. Cath answered promptly that at Gerry and Susan's school, children often went out for 'appointments'. Mark interrupted, 'I want one of them, too!' Smiling, I replied that it sounded like they could *all* say they had an appointment, or they could tell the other children they had special time in a playroom, if they wanted to. We would plan for them to come eight times, and then see if more times would be a good idea or not. Mark shouted 'more, more'. I smiled, replying that Mark was sure already that he wanted more. We would have eight times and then maybe more.

Before I left I said that their social worker, John, would be asking me what I thought each one of them needed after I got to know them better in my playroom. I knew that they were not seeing their Mum and Dad right now, and the judge in court needed to hear what I said about that too. The judge would listen to John and me, their Mum and Dad, and other people to make up his mind about the children seeing their parents. I'd go once to see their Mum and Dad too. I added that John had told me about how Mark had been hurt while his Mum and Dad had been taking care of him and about how they had all come to live with Cath and Edward. The three children looked very anxious as I talked, with even Mark becoming very subdued. I said it was hard for them to hear about all these things and that was all I needed to say to them. Maybe they wanted to say something to me or ask me about something? But if not, Cath would be able to talk more about everything I had said to them – it was a lot of new things to remember.

Meeting the children's parents

My meeting with the children's parents took place at their nearest family centre. I had written to them, explaining who I was, and that I had been asked by social services to begin play therapy sessions and later to prepare a report for the court on their children's needs, wishes and feelings towards contact with them. I hoped to meet them to introduce myself, to explain to them as the children's parents how I planned to try to help their children and to answer any questions they might have about my work. I added that I would also be interested in what they thought their children needed from them as parents.

In the event the meeting proved a difficult one, and productive only perhaps in giving me first-hand experience of the children's parents. Mr and Mrs Seaton vehemently expressed their anger with social services and the court for their children's Care Order, their feeling that nobody understood how difficult their children were, how they hadn't ever had any help with them from social services and how they hadn't done anything to hurt the children in any way. Having acknowledged their feelings, I tried to direct the conversation onto the children's past histories and their parents' methods of child care, but Mr Seaton persisted in maintaining that everything had been fine, except for the children being 'downright wicked' sometimes. Mr Seaton volunteered when I asked for more details that the children all got up to 'tricks' and ended up falling down or starting to light into one another. I asked how he comforted his children when they did get hurt, and perhaps did each child need different things at different times? Mr Seaton was firmly of the opinion that on the contrary, all they needed was picking up and a plaster put on when hurt, and keeping apart when fighting. Neither Mr nor Mrs Seaton wanted to recall or relate any particular incident. Mrs Seaton said she couldn't remember very well, that she tried not to think about the past because it was too painful to then come back to the present and face not having the children with her. I suggested that from what they'd just said maybe it was easier to think about their more recent visits with the children.

As they were beginning to become impatient with me, saying that I was asking too many questions, I suggested that they might like to know about my method of non-directive play therapy, trying to explain, in the face of their strongly worded disapproval, that although I wouldn't allow the children to hurt themselves or me or damage property, there would be toys for children of different ages in the room and the children were allowed to talk about and play with whatever they wanted. Mrs Seaton asked if Gerry was going to play with baby toys, then! I replied that older children did sometimes choose to play with toys for younger children, especially when they were remembering events from their past or when they had younger emotions to express. Mrs Seaton, backed by Mr Seaton, asked querulously whether they could do just *anything* then. I replied that many parents and carers asked me that same question. I thought it was a good one and that I was careful to show children that there were rules in the playroom, even though there weren't so many of them, and that children understood that they were able to have more freedom in the 'special time' with me in the playroom than in school or at home.

They became even more irate when I indicated that I would be audio recording my sessions with the children, and that I had been asked to submit a report to the court. I acknowledged their frustration and resentment in not being able to change the way I worked. I could only reassure them that my tapes and notes would remain confidential, outside of legal matters and progress reports to social services. Although these brief reports would be for social services' use, they might wish to contact the children's social worker at his office if they wanted more information.

I listened again to their grievances against social services on the way downstairs, and answered when they paused a moment that it would be a shame for their children if their parents were on one side and felt everyone else connected with the children were against them. Their children could feel caught in the middle of a battle. Mr and Mrs Seaton decided to have the last word, shouting back to me on their way out of the door that *they* were willing to forget about everything that had been done to them as long as they got their children back. I returned to the family room, feeling somewhat wrung out and irritable, decided to make myself a drink and apologise to the secretary for the parents' noisy parting. I then spent some time quietly reflecting on what the children themselves, rather than I, might feel about their parents.

SUSAN'S FIRST PLAY THERAPY SESSION

Susan began her first session by bursting into the room, having waited in the other playroom with Cath and Gerry while Mark had the first session with me. After running around the room randomly for a short time, she chose a small hammer and workbench, pounding the pegs noisily and haphazardly. Without looking up from pounding, she asked, 'Did Mark do this?' and 'What's this for?' Hearing the urgency in her voice and responding to this tone, I replied, 'You want to know why you're here and what to do'. Susan did not answer, but became very still and alert, looking down at the pegs in front of her. Using simple sentence structures and vocabulary, I explained briefly that this was Susan's special time and she could do what she wanted. Mark could tell Susan about what he had done if he wanted, and she could talk to anybody she wanted about anything we did. I wouldn't talk much about it to anybody. But I would have to tell John and the judge what she needed. Susan glanced at me briefly, remaining still.

I showed her the tape and explained how I would use it while Susan returned to her pounding. After a rapid flurry of activity, she ran over to return the workbench and hammer to the shelf, then ran over to the play telephone box. Without slowing down, she hurried to me with one of the two toy telephones she had found, returned to the telephone box and went through the motions of a pretend telephone call to me. This telephoning was done in a rudimentary manner, with Susan seemingly more interested in the process of telephoning and finding the numbers on the dial than in engaging in a conversation. After a brief time, she emerged from the phone box giggling. Focusing on her feelings, I commented, 'That was fun!'

She then turned rapidly to painting and asked for a big paper 'like Mark's'. I responded that Susan wanted to be sure to be the same as Mark. Holding a large brush between her thumb and other fingers in a fist, she filled the entire paper with different colours, while she and I talked about this process – how Susan didn't like too much paint at once, but couldn't take it off again, and how she liked all the different colours, and so on. After filling the paper with an overlay of several colours, she handed me her painting. She noticed paint on the counter and hastily tried to clean it up. I remarked that Susan was worried; she did not want it to be messy. Susan did not reply, but asked for another paper, this time deciding it would be different from Mark's. I briefly added, 'What *you* want to do this time'. Looking again at the paint remaining on the table, Susan remarked, 'We need to wipe it up'. Noting her use of 'we', I immediately offered to help Susan because 'you don't want it to be messy'. Susan decided, 'You do it', and started her next painting. While she painted this time, she talked about going to the telephone box after she finished painting, about wanting to paint a house and about how she would stay for a long time. I replied that Susan seemed to want to be in the playroom for a long time, doing lots of things. The conversation continued:

> V: Maybe it seemed like a long time to wait to come in here.
> Susan nodded vigorously while she painted.
> V: Maybe you didn't want to wait.
> S: No, I didn't want to.

> V: Now you have a long time here by yourself.
> S: I'm going to do lots of painting.
> V: Lots. You like it.

Susan talked about the house she was painting but then moved over to the finger paints without completing it. Dipping her finger in, she worried about whether the paint would come off. Reassured by me that it would clean off, Susan again referred to her younger brother, asking whether he had used these paints. I once again explained that children could talk about what they did in the playroom if they wanted to, but that I myself tried not to, unless I had to tell a judge or a social worker what the children needed.

> V: Maybe you were waiting and waiting and wondering what Mark was doing up here.
> S: Maybe this. Painting.
> V: Maybe the same as you.

Susan then opened all the containers of finger paints, taking big blobs out and smearing them all over her hands somewhat frantically. She stopped suddenly, becoming worried about whether the paint would come off her hands, and became even more agitated when she saw paint on the floor. I reassured her that it was all right to get paint on the floor at that end of the room, and that the tiles could be cleaned up. Susan then piled very large amounts of finger paints onto her paper, while I commented that she liked to get very messy, but she also needed to be sure it could be cleaned up.

Susan smeared the paint on the paper for a while, paused and playfully went towards my face with her paint-covered hands, looking directly at me and giggling. I said, smiling, 'You're teasing. You want to put it on my face'. Susan then tentatively touched her own face with her painted hands.

> V: You're not sure that it's allowed. You can do it if you like.
> S: Can children do what they like?
> V: They can be messy here, but not over there. We can't clean it off the rug and chairs. It looks like you want to put it on your face. There's a mirror over there if you want it.

She went to the mirror and giggled as she looked in the mirror, putting paint on her nose and quickly wiping it off again. I remarked that Susan liked paint on, but then wanted it off right away. Susan then painted different colours on her face, saying, 'I'm going downstairs like this'.

> V: Everybody has to get clean before they leave. When they're in the playroom, they can be messy and do mostly what they like, but then get cleaned up at the end.

S: Why?
V: Because it's a special time in here to do what you want. But not downstairs and outside. Everything stays here, except what you make and want to take home.

Susan smeared paint around her face, smiling broadly into the mirror and stroking her face enthusiastically. I warned her to mind her eyes, but was unable to stop Susan inadvertently rubbing a bit into one of her eyes.

S: [very softly] Ooh.
V: [in a concerned tone] Is it stinging your eye? Does it hurt? I can't tell.
Susan moaned slightly.
V: I'm trying to take care of you. I didn't think the paints could sting you. Maybe I can help you get it out of your eye.

Susan made a small non-verbal motion that she wanted me to help her. While working at dabbing Susan's eye, I commented that Susan *did* want to be messy, but now she needed help for her eye to feel better. Susan remained impassive and silent as she accepted my assistance.

V: Maybe next time the face paints and not the finger paints will be better to use.
[Susan nodded]
V: I get worried when that stings. I don't want you to get hurt.

After her face was clean, Susan began to tidy up the paints, stopped and returned to the play telephone box. This time she felt confident enough to tell me not to give her hard numbers to dial and we had a conversation, led by Susan, about her getting paint in her eye.

V: It worried you a bit.
S: Yeah, and then you helped me, didn't ya?
V: Yes, I didn't want you to get hurt. You're pleased I helped you. . . . It's almost time to go now.

Susan rang me again on the telephone with the message she wanted to stay.

V: Yes, I know you do. You can come back next time. It's going to be Gerry's turn now.
S: Not now. Not yet.
V: It's hard to leave. There's so much to play with. It's almost time to go now. The clock over there on the wall is pointing to almost three o'clock. I'll wait for you to have one more go on the telephone before we leave.

Susan had a brief dial and then left the room easily, walking with me and chatting eagerly. On the way downstairs, Susan confided that she knew Mark had been naughty and had made a mess. I replied that children could be messy in the playroom with me and not get into trouble. After saying goodbye to Susan, I said I would fix up the room for Gerry and return to get him shortly.

SUSAN'S THERAPEUTIC PROGRESS

Several themes emerged in Susan's first session and were worked through and developed subsequently. By identifying these, and then tracing changes in her play which occurred in later sessions, it is possible to demonstrate her therapeutic progress.

Several features of Susan's first and subsequent sessions supported the hypothesis that her emotional difficulties arose as a consequence of physical abuse, making it necessary for her to make unhealthy adaptations in order to survive. In her first session, Susan found the non-directive nature of her play sessions difficult to utilise, partly owing to her inability to stimulate herself or to concentrate on activities for more than short periods of time, but also because of her anxiety over being messy, and her fear of adult anger and disapproval. She often attempted to imitate her brothers in an effort to avoid making mistakes and being blamed herself, and needed to receive the therapist's reassurance and permission before attempting an activity herself. Another notable feature of the first session was her passivity when her eye was stinging. She was unable to express her distress, to the point that the therapist needed to ask her if she was hurt.

Her emotional conflicts in the first sessions centred first on sharing the therapist and playroom with her two brothers. She seemed to need more time for herself, a need probably derived from her parents' inability to fulfil their children's needs because their own were overriding. Second, on her exploration of materials and her messiness, which was in conflict with her eagerness to tidy up and thus please adults. After her first session, Susan's messiness increasingly involved an element of defiance towards an adult, the therapist, as well as an element of disliking herself. In motor activities in particular, Susan painted or drew haphazardly and impulsively, and commonly ended this type of activity by making a mess. This messiness led in turn to great frustration with herself as she unsuccessfully attempted to clean up, needing to have an adult help her and then resenting her dependence on that adult.

She expressed these themes in various ways throughout her early and middle sessions. By the middle sessions, she was defiantly making messes with paints in the sink, on the floor and on the table for the therapist to clean up. She also gradually began to devise role-plays of adult–child situations, with the therapist in the role of the naughty girl and Susan in the role of the powerful, merciless adult in authority.

As her therapy progressed, Susan moved from being unable to settle to any activity during the hour to discovering meaningful games and play patterns for herself. Her capacity to concentrate on activities she had chosen, to return to these activities following distractions and to persist with them despite frustrations increased markedly. There were also less emotion-laden sequences of play, in which Susan played shops, while the therapist's role, given to her by Susan, was to be a customer and admire her goods. (See Chapter 2 on Patrick for a discussion of the development of the capacity for symbolic play.)

In her later therapy sessions, Susan began to enact role-plays, with dolls in the roles of children and herself as either a good or bad mother, or the therapist in the role of the bad mother; the children were themselves abandoned or harmed. These role-plays were powerful enactments of deep-seated, painful and conflicting emotions which she experienced towards herself, her siblings and her mother, and which she was able to re-experience and re-examine within the playroom. Through these role-plays, Susan was able to re-integrate her relatively permanent personal schemas towards her mother on motor, cognitive and affective levels of functioning, resulting in a re-alignment of her personality.

This change was demonstrated in all areas of her life; her school work improved and her foster carers reported greater assertiveness, initiative and playfulness at home. Her change in attitude was also demonstrated clearly in one of her final therapy sessions, in which she decided to make playdough hearts, one for her foster carer, Cath, and one for her mother. After working on the first shape and completing it successfully, she began to make one for her mother. This one 'went wrong' and Susan decided to throw it away and put it readily into the waste paper basket. She did not, as she would have done previously, need to make a defiant mess, become angry with herself, or need to destroy her other model. The negative emotions she felt towards her mother seemed clarified and focused, so that she would be more able to proceed with normal development.

These therapeutic gains were supported by skilled foster care and the close involvement of the children's social worker, John. Four years later, despite some set-backs for her brothers, Susan is still doing well in the same foster home.

THEORETICAL ISSUE

Underlying assumptions of non-directive play therapy

We turn now to the theoretical underpinnings of non-directive play therapy and the ways that these principles were realised in Susan's sessions. It will be evident in the following discussion that some of the theoretical issues in later chapters are relevant to Susan's case, most notably our theoretical discussion of physical abuse in Chapter 4.

Susan's first session illustrates the key features of non-directive play therapy. In the first session, the therapist helps the child to understand the uniqueness of the therapeutic environment: that the focus is on the child, not on the therapist, and the therapist's focus is primarily on the child's feelings; that the child rather than the therapist chooses the pace and contents of the sessions; that there is a permissive atmosphere, although some rules still apply; and that the therapist's role is to help the child and to respond quickly and appropriately to the child's needs. Each of these principles of non-directive play therapy will be illustrated below using Susan's first session.

Other therapeutic approaches utilise some of these principles, forming the basis for a new *rapprochement* among non-directive, object relation and interpersonal relationship theorists on the importance of allowing the child to develop an immediate relationship with the therapist (Heard and Lake, 1986; Chethick, 1989; Bacal and Newman, 1990; Zeanah et al., 1990; Wilson et al., 1992). Some therapists within the psychoanalytic tradition seek to minimise interpretation to children in briefer therapeutic encounters (Bettelheim and Rosenfeld, 1993; Judd, 1993). (See also our further discussion of interpretation from a non-directive perspective in Chapter 7.) Bettelheim in discussing milieu therapy, for example, advocates that '. . . in child therapy, the interpretation usually ought to stay within the displacement . . . talking about what the toy doll did, not about what the action means in the child patient's own life and family. If we do make a direct interpretation to a child, it can feel very intrusive, make the child anxious and lead him or her to change the subject' (1993: 162).

The development of a trusting, accepting relationship between the therapist and the child

Creating a trusting environment for troubled and abused children is necessarily more difficult because of their previous disturbed relationships with adults. Susan, like many other children, was initially uneasy in an unknown situation, although this anxiety was alleviated somewhat by having her brothers and foster carer nearby. The therapist consciously sensed Susan's unease and responded to this by speaking to her in a quiet voice, avoiding direct eye contact, except very briefly, allowing Susan to maintain a comfortable (to Susan) physical distance between them and giving her brief facts at the beginning to help her understand this new experience. Susan's feeling of trust in the therapist and trust in herself developed during the session, particularly when the therapist showed concern at the paint stinging her eye. Afterwards, Susan directed the conversation back to the incident, consciously thinking about this experience and about her feeling of developing trust in the therapist.

The acceptance by the therapist that the child chooses the focus of activity

With abused and troubled children, a vital aspect of therapy is the re-establishment of choice and autonomy (Wilson et al., 1992; Ryan, 1995a; Ryan and Wilson, 1995a). Sometimes this choice begins at the rudimentary level of the therapist allowing the child to express feelings which are different and often in direct conflict with the therapist's feelings and wishes, for example, Susan's wish for more time at the end of her session. The child's oppositional and negative feelings may be expressed directly, without the child feeling punished or rejected by the therapist for this negativity. This wilfulness of a child in play therapy is very similar to a one- to two-year-old child beginning to learn that he or she has some autonomy in regulating his/her life, that choices do not lie only with the carers. Negative and oppositional choices are the clearest and most rudimentary forms of autonomy and are the basis for the beginning of a child's growth of identity and self-determination (Erikson, 1963). An abused or traumatised child needs to learn that any situation that is emotionally painful which he or she experiences or remembers does not have to be dealt with in a passive, resistant, powerless way. By taking an active stance within therapy and within his or her own thoughts about a situation, the child turns a passive stance into a self-determining one. Recent research on resilient individuals who have remained emotionally healthy despite adverse life conditions, such as adolescents whose mothers were suffering from depressive illnesses (Beardsley, 1991), suggests that their resilience involves taking an active stance towards these problems.

In non-directive play therapy a child is given genuine choices of activities and conversations and is able actively to choose the medium that best expresses his or her personality and emotional responses. In Susan's case, she had great difficulty in her initial sessions in maintaining her own independent focus for her activities. She rapidly shifted from one activity to another in a disorganised and somewhat chaotic way. But because the therapist established a permissive atmosphere and allowed her to direct her own actions, she was able to explore her environment and her thoughts and feelings independently from her brothers, in ways which seemed likely to have been previously greatly curtailed. She actively assimilated her discomfort over her eye and chose to think about the therapist's response to her feeling of pain in this incident.

The reflection of the child's feelings by the therapist in a non-threatening manner

In non-directive play therapy, the therapist listens, recognises and responds to a child's feelings in order to help the child towards greater self-awareness. When these feelings and actions are expressed within a trusting relationship, it is assumed that these feelings will lose much of their negative power. In Susan's initial session, for example, her undue anxiety emerged about the need to be tidy while simultaneously strongly wishing to explore in messy ways. The therapist joined these two conflicting feelings together verbally for Susan as she experienced them. The therapist did not, however, link the feeling of being bad with being messy and the feeling of being good with being tidy, nor did she link these conflicting feelings with Susan's mother or father because Susan herself had not consciously made these links. It was only at the end of the session that Susan began to address her emotional schema of bad being equated with messiness by referring to her brother – not, it should be noted, to herself – as being naughty. The therapist kept Susan's referrant, and broadened it to the more general concept of 'children', rather than personalising it in a way which Susan might have found emotionally too threatening.

In non-directive play therapy the therapist, rather than interpreting the child's behaviour or addressing the child's coping (defence) mechanisms directly, instead has the child freely assimilate his or her mental activity in a non-threatening environment. The therapist attempts to help the child make conscious and give symbolic representation to thoughts which are largely outside conscious awareness. The child's problems are dealt with on a symbolic level, which includes discussing the child's feelings and thoughts directly when the child wishes to do so. The therapist herself does not actively initiate solutions to the child's real life problems within therapy (see Wilson et al. 1992 for a fuller discussion). It is assumed that this kind of approach will help a child to deal both internally and externally with his or her current and future life experiences. That is, 'One of the most characteristic and perhaps one of the most important changes in therapy is the bringing into awareness of experiences of which heretofore the child has not been conscious' (Rogers, 1976: 147).

With the therapist's accurate verbal reflection and appropriate non-verbal responses to Susan's conflicting feelings, it is assumed that Susan will be enabled to alter, abandon and/or integrate her existing, incompatible mental schemas. It should again be noted that the therapist *does* interpret the material of Susan's session to herself. As we discuss further in the final chapter, therapeutic interpretation and developmental assessment are an essential part of the therapist's role, and enable her to reflect feelings accurately as well as to assess the child's therapeutic progress.

The establishment of appropriate therapeutic boundaries

As we state in our earlier book: 'The guiding principles for the use of limits in non-directive therapy are that they both should reflect the practical reality of the constraints imposed by the physical context in which the therapy is conducted, and should also address the therapeutic needs of the child. In relation to the latter, the skill needed is to establish a level of permissiveness which is sufficient to allow the child to express and explore feelings freely, and at the same time to set boundaries to the child's behaviour which will both offer a sense of security and the potential for certain therapeutic experiences' (1992: 205).

Susan's first session enabled the therapist to set out many of the usual therapeutic limits for the use of the room, confidentiality and the amount of time for the session. Rather than the therapist listing these limits at the outset, the rules arose within the context of therapy itself, made sense for Susan by their immediacy, and addressed Susan's emotional needs for safety and security. Susan's emotional needs were both acknowledged overtly and met by the therapist's manner of enforcing limits, for example, by saying that the hour was finished, while at the same time recognising and helping Susan to make conscious for herself her oppositional feelings of not having enough from the hour and wanting more time.

PRACTICE ISSUES

Working therapeutically with children in a statutory setting

In this section we address practice concerns which are specific to working therapeutically with children in a statutory setting. We also touch on more general practice issues in the first stages of therapy. Our underlying position in this and later sections on practice is that a practitioner's understanding of theory and research continually interacts with practice. In our discussion, therefore, we try to show how theoretical material and research findings inform the therapist's hypotheses and decisions.

A general practice issue at referral is the danger that the therapist's view of the child will be coloured in advance by other professional's opinions (Wilson et al., 1992). For this reason, some child therapists (e.g. Bettelheim and Rosenfeld, 1993) advise beginning therapists in particular to refrain from reading records or discussing the case with other professionals before they themselves have been able to experience the child in an unprejudiced and personal way. Because the child is unknown to them, potentially difficult and unresponsive to help, at this stage therapists may make strenuous attempts to allay their heightened anxiety. By eschewing information, therapists will guard against being unduly influenced by the judgments of authoritative professionals.

Although this argument is persuasive, we would argue, as a later chapter on a boy with multiple medical, attachment and abuse-related problems shows (see Delroy, Chapter 5), that the therapist's anxiety can at times be greater when she has underestimated the severity of the child's problems and not had, arguably, enough information at referral. Our position, therefore, is that the therapists need to have training, supervision and self-discipline to guard themselves against *both* types of mistakes as much as possible.

Assessment of the child's current environment and care plan

One of the therapist's first concerns at Susan's referral was whether she would benefit from non-directive play therapy sessions. Her problems did not seem too severe for intervention on a weekly basis. Susan was managing to function, although at the lowest ability level, within mainstream schooling and neither her carers nor her teachers found her behaviour unmanageable. With some other referred cases, however, the child's behaviour may be very dangerous and destructive to himself or to others, and outside the control of adult authority; or the child's behaviour and thought may display bizarre and fragmented patterns, as in conditions such as autism (Frith, 1989) or hyperactivity (Weiss and Hechtman, 1986). These and other reactions in children may be due to a physical and/or psychiatric condition, or to unknown severe abuse and would warrant a psychiatric assessment. In these cases intensive psychiatric or psychotherapeutic involvement may be necessary, rather than weekly play therapy sessions. (Again, see Chapter 5, Delroy, for a child with more serious problems of this type.) Other conditions may appear to be primarily physical and further medical information from a paediatric assessment should be sought; the therapist will have to keep in mind, of course, the possibility of a physical basis for any unusual behaviour by a child throughout her work.

A further consideration at referral is whether the child's carers, either foster carers or natural parents, provide an at least minimally acceptable environment in which the child can change and develop. Weekly play therapy sessions rely for their effectiveness on the child being able to work through emotional experiences and attitudes which have emerged during therapy, and to try out new and more effective behaviours in everyday life outside of therapy. If the child's environment is not adequate, this is the first and most important area to address, rather than beginning with therapeutic help (Wolff, 1989; Glaser, 1992). With children in foster placements, the reasons for their being received into care necessarily involve some degree of disruption or loss of permanent parenting figures. Therapists need to be cautious in attributing all of the child's emotional problems to past trauma, or as in Susan's case, to past and recurring trauma due to her parents' visits. Court proceedings, which can often be lengthy and inconclusive, and disruptions in foster placements can also contribute significantly to a child's emotional instability. In addition, a therapist must also consider the possibility that emotional difficulties of children in foster care may be due to their current care. As we highlight in other chapters, the fact that the child's environment must provide a certain level of support in order for therapy to be effective. In addition, as our discussion on the role of foster carers below demonstrates, the child's carers have a vital role to play in a child's therapeutic change. This needs to be seen very much as a joint enterprise.

Susan's foster home emerged at referral as providing her with a highly nurturing atmosphere. The foster carers' attitudes towards all three children were strongly positive ones, and they expressed throughout our meetings feelings of concern, warmth and intelligent flexibility towards the children, which included adapting quickly to the increased demands on their time and emotional energy required by play therapy. Susan's home environment and care plan, then, appeared satisfactory and stable enough to allow her the emotional resources she would need in her therapy sessions and in her everyday life to benefit from play therapy, even though her future was subject to court proceedings.

Consideration of alternative therapies

However, perhaps another form of intervention, such as family or group therapy would be more appropriate than individual sessions? John, as the social worker, had already concluded that family sessions were inappropriate. This decision seemed valid, given the non-cooperation of the parents and their inability to take responsibility for their own behaviour (Wilson and Ryan, 1994). Temporary termination of the parents' contact with their children because of the children's emotional distress, as well as a care plan which was now moving towards a permanent placement with a Residence Order for the children, also argued strongly against this option.

Other possibilities to consider were whether joint sessions with all three siblings or a therapeutic group for physically abused children (if such a group existed in the area) would be more appropriate than individual therapy (Dwivedi, 1993). Several features of Susan's and her brothers' behaviour seemed to argue against these group approaches. First, the therapist was influenced by the known effects on children of an abusive environment (discussed further in chapter 3). This research implied that

Susan's emotional responses of tearfulness and overcompliance, her developmental delay and poor intellectual functioning were probably longstanding adaptations to abusive parenting. The therapist noted that Susan seemed unable to relinquish these previous adaptations after many months in a nurturing environment, which further underlined the serious effects of her earlier lengthy neglect by her parents. An intensive environment with play therapy sessions focusing on individual child–adult interactions thus seemed highly appropriate (see chapter 2 for more details of this argument).

Second, Cath's examples of the day-to-day interactions of the three children in the household showed an intense rivalry between Gerry and Mark for the exclusive attention of their foster carers. Susan was said to react to this rivalry by withdrawal and passivity, or tearful outbursts and clinging to Cath, behaviours which remained unchanged despite Cath's appropriate responses to them. Again, these factors seemed to argue for a more intensive intervention for each child, as well as confirming that a lower intensity intervention, such as the therapist offering consultations with the children's carers and social worker, would not suffice.

An added question at referral with Susan, because of her educational difficulties but not with her brothers, was whether a non-directive approach was appropriate for her problems. Some educational and child psychologists would argue that because Susan's educational assessment showed an inability to concentrate and high impulsivity, a highly structured environment with activities directed by the adult was warranted, rather than an approach in which the child herself chooses the focus of activity.

The arguments for non-directive play therapy for Susan seemed nonetheless stronger. Apart from the fact that Susan was already receiving this type of educational input at her school, the permissive atmosphere of a non-directive approach is often misunderstood by professionals working with children. In particular, it is in crucial ways a highly structured approach when practised as an overall method (see Wilson et al., 1992). A further argument for using a non-directive approach with Susan was that studies on resilient individuals and the development of competence, mentioned above, demonstrate that children and adults need to develop an internal stand and internal locus of control over their actions in order to function effectively. Non-directive play therapy, by focusing on the child's freedom of choice within a structured environment, provides such a learning situation. Finally, an additional argument in Susan's case was that her intellectual functioning and impulsivity seemed to be highly influenced by her emotional difficulties, as her educational assessment stated. A therapeutic approach concentrating on her emotional life, therefore, seemed desirable.

Although concluding that individual play therapy was appropriate for Susan and her brothers, the therapist also recognised the importance of their relationships to one another (Dunn and Kendrick, 1982; Dunn and McGuire, 1992; Cohen, 1993). Unfortunately, although joint sessions with all three children together towards the end of their individual sessions might have been indicated, financial constraints made it unlikely that funding for these would be available, given that the children's primary relationship problems seemed entrenched and would take a significant amount of time to be resolved. In addition, Susan's educational assessment indicated that she might have low intellectual ability in addition to her emotional problems, which could make therapeutic progress slower for her than for her brothers. However, the possibility would be kept in mind by the therapist throughout her individual work. It might also be possible to extend the children's funding through the therapist's recommendations to the court, if this seemed needed when she came to write her report.

To offset this lack of attention to interactions among the children in their individual sessions, the therapist was encouraged that Susan and her brothers would potentially benefit from the more intensive interactions they had with Cath during the time they were waiting for their sessions. It should be recognised that sometimes by providing children with regularly occurring intensive sessions, other new relationships or intensifications of old relationships also become possible (Wilson et al., 1992). Susan and her brothers would have more exclusive attention, shared with only one other sibling, from Cath during their waiting time. Like the play therapy room, the room they wait in was another well-equipped playroom in the same building, also free from outside interruptions. These conditions were similar to some of the conditions for non-directive filial therapy (Guerney, 1984; van Fleet, 1994) in which the carer is the primary therapist and receives supervision from a trained therapist. Although Cath did not receive intensive supervision, the therapist did make general suggestions and give more specific guidance at times in ways she could help the children understand what they were thinking and feeling in a free play situation. Since Cath herself had already developed this attitude of paying close attention to the children's emotions and helping them to express their feelings, the therapist's suggestions were a natural extension of Cath's general approach. In other cases much more input and monitoring of the carer's responses to the child by other professionals may be needed in order to help the carer respond therapeutically, which we will discuss next.

Foster carers and play therapy

As we have seen, foster carers have an essential role to play in non-directive play therapy. Rather than the therapist in any sense usurping the carer's role, the therapist needs to make the foster carer into an active participant in the therapeutic process. Indeed, signs that the child is more attached to the therapist rather than the carer should give rise to concerns about either the adequacy of the child's environment or the appropriateness of the therapeutic relationship itself. It is also damaging to the child's relationship with a carer for the therapist to promise either the alleviation of symptoms which the carer considers to be a problem or a child's steady, uncomplicated progress, both of which are outside of the therapist's (or anyone's!) exclusive control. Foster carers and social workers have realistically to expect more demands on their time, thinking and emotional energy while therapy is taking place. The therapist also needs to be persuasive and sensitive to these professonals' initial reluctance to fulfil this function, however committed to the child's welfare they are, because their professional lives are often already overly demanding, as Delroy's story in chapter 5 vividly illustrates.

Another feature of the pivotal role of the child's carer is the therapist's dependence on the carer to provide her with precise current information on the child's emotional functioning. For example, the therapist needed specifically to ask Cath for details of incidents and behaviours at their referral meeting, rather than relying on more general descriptions such as 'competitive' or 'clinging'. As their meeting continued, both Cath and John became more precise as they began to appreciate the level of description useful to the therapist. Foster carers are also asked as part of their role to keep daily event or incident diaries with the children in their care. These diaries in the authors' experience are often an under-rated source of information on the child, as are foster carers' verbal accounts. Only minimal training is given if at all to carers or to professional staff in residential care settings, in keeping objective, accurate records. When the therapist has these more detailed descriptions rather than generalised accounts and interpretations, she is able more accurately and thoroughly to consider reasons for the children's behaviour herself.

The play therapist should also be aware of other general issues in working with foster carers. Similarly to the child's natural parents, the foster carer requires adequate information on the method of therapeutic intervention itself, the possible effects on a child outside of sessions and the child's need for some degree of privacy to work through emotionally difficult experiences. However, the foster carer's role *is* different from a parent's role with a child (Fahlberg, 1988). Foster carers do not have a shared life history or usually as close an identification with the child as the child's natural parents. There are, of course, exceptions: some foster carers decide to foster because of their own personal histories of abandonment, lack of love or abuse which they have not thoroughly and consciously come to accept on an adult level (Fahlberg, 1986). Under these circumstances the foster carer may identify strongly with the child and in rare cases may actively abuse a child. The therapist must always be alert to this possibility and be aware that all the difficulties which can arise with abusive parents, such as trying to keep the child from betraying the family's secrets, resulting in being potentially hazardous for the child, could then apply. In general, though, foster carers are likely to be more free of certain emotionally difficult reactions which natural parents may have to play therapy, such as fear of criticism or a need to block the child's therapeutic progress in order to maintain the status quo in the family.

While foster carers may not be as prone to intense emotional reactions when a child in their care begins play therapy, certain other concerns may arise. Clearly they wish the child to be introduced to a professional whom they themselves consider to be trustworthy and competent. However, current training and the support systems of foster leaders and/or other professional foster carers, whether organised or *ad hoc*, is at the moment unlikely to given them much guidance on their role in therapeutic work. Because most foster carers are aware of the increased emotional vulnerability of a child due to being in care, they may have understandable reservations about helping a child begin an intervention unfamiliar to them with an unknown professional. Yet because of their own lower level of training compared with that of the therapist, they may feel intimidated and unable to express these concerns openly.

A foster carer may also be concerned that they are unequal to the task outlined by the therapist. Since no airtight guarantee of therapeutic progress can be given by the therapist at referral, the carers may fear that the child's behaviour could deteriorate and their already demanding relationship with the child will become impossible to maintain. Instead of readily participating in the therapeutic process as active participants with the child and therapist then, foster carers may gravitate towards the role of passive observers themselves, while the therapist 'fixes' the child. Another reason for passive or unhelpful reactions, rather than active participation by foster carers, may be that they have already felt overwhelmed emotionally in caring for the child. If, for instance, they have struggled with what they perceive as inadequate professional and personal support in dealing with a child's difficult behaviour over a period of time, they may want to abdicate their carer's role to the therapist, at least to some degree.

Carers seem particularly vulnerable to abdication when they have felt burdened by the child's continuing negativity and unhappiness, and have come to feel a sense of despair and hopelessness themselves about the child's future. While the carers' attitude may be an unconscious reflection of the child's own attitude towards him or herself, it may also be based on direct or unconscious emotional messages from other key professionals for the child. However, the play therapy referral itself conveys the equally powerful counter-message to carers that the therapist and other child care professionals are hopeful that the child can be restored to a normal developmental pathway. An extra resource and extra attention is now being made available to the child.

For all these reasons the play therapist needs to explore the carers' attitudes towards play therapy at referral and allow them to form a personal opinion of the method and of the therapist herself. She also needs to place in perspective the carers' own role in relation to herself and the social worker, and to be aware of the carers' ongoing support system. It is often helpful for the therapist to discuss explicitly how the foster carers can best respond to the child about therapy, in keeping with a non-directive approach. Key areas the therapist should cover are that the child needs them to show general interest in the child's well-being and an openness to any communications the child might choose to reveal, as well as a heightened responsiveness to the child's feelings and behaviour. These points then need to be illustrated using concrete examples. It is helpful to the child when carers recognise the permissiveness of the playroom and that some of the rules of polite behaviour need not apply, e.g. 'You're not saying "good-bye" properly' or 'Be a good girl in there'. The therapist can also explain that it is not useful for the child if they are too inquisitive, e.g. 'Tell me all about what you and Virginia did today' or too directive, e.g. 'Be sure to make me a picture in the playroom'.

The play therapist should also emphasise to the foster carers her own dependence on the social worker's role, which is to offer support and advice to carers on general therapeutic issues. The social worker will have a general familiarity with the aims of therapy from his own training and will also be experienced in supporting the foster carer in dealing with the child's general behaviour. More specific issues directly related to therapeutic contents may also arise, including the social worker helping foster carers distinguish the behaviour of the child's which is related to therapy from other behaviours. Support may also have to be given by the social worker for carers to maintain reasonable boundaries to the child's behaviour, while remaining flexible and able to incorporate changes into the child's established patterns of response. In Susan's case, John talked with Cath about the increased messiness Susan showed at home during her early sessions and worked out with Cath how boundaries could be maintained in the home. He also helped Cath to designate a place in the kitchen for messier activities which could easily be cleaned up afterwards.

Foster carers usually respond favourably and actively to the possibility of play therapy for a troubled child they care for and feel relief and a sense of effectiveness, as Cath did, that they are being listened to about the emotional needs they perceive in their foster child. Very occasionally, carers may become more rigid and unable to listen to others' opinions who do not share the same job. More commonly, however, as foster carers gain more experience with children attending play therapy, they become more confident with therapists and other professionals, more able to ask questions and receive desired information, and more adept at giving detailed information spontaneously to the therapist on the child.

Introductory meetings

We shall mention practice considerations in meeting a child's parents in a statutory setting where the child no longer lives at home only briefly here, since we refer to these issues again in the last chapter of this book in relation to court proceedings. The section then considers practice issues for the therapist in introductory visits before discussing the final practice issue of the chapter, the therapist's attitude of 'free-floating attention' during play therapy sessions.

Introductory meetings with parents

In many circumstances within a statutory setting where the child's parents are working in cooperation with social services for their child's best interests, it is helpful for the social worker to introduce the therapist to the child's parents. The social worker's role, as we have stated above, is to work with parents, helping them to implement changes in their parental functioning. S/he would also then be more able to explain play therapy further to them as questions arose in the course of their child's intervention, and a joint meeting may be viewed by the social worker as a useful opportunity to emphasise and hear the therapist give added weight to facets of his or her own ongoing supportive or rehabilitative work with the child's parents.

Sometimes, however, the therapist may choose to have separate meetings initially with the child's parents. Her status as an independent professional enables parents to discuss their children from their own perspective more readily. The therapist will then also be able to form her opinions of the parents based on her own separate observations and interactions with them, rather than their meeting being strongly biased by the social worker's and parents' relationship with one another.

In our earlier book and again in the last chapter of this book we have emphasised that conducting non-directive play therapy sessions or assessments with a child who is living in an abusive environment can be a source of physical danger or psychological harm to the child, and should be avoided. With children who are not living at home but whose parents or carers have been abusive, as in Susan's case, supervised contact visits themselves may be times in which parents continue to be abusive or still to exert subtler forms of coercion or direct threats which are emotionally harmful to the child. This type of emotional harm is difficult for supervising staff to detect and prevent. Both the therapist during her sessional work and other workers with the child need to be alert to the possibility that parents who are hostile to their child's therapy because of their own fear of criminal charges or loss of their children may deliberately attempt to undermine the therapist's work with the child. With Susan and her brothers these risks in participating in individual therapy no longer applied, since contact had been suspended. In the therapist's meeting with their parents, however, there were indications that they might have tried to control or unduly influence their children's behaviour during their therapy sessions, given the opportunity.

It was important, however, that the therapist meet with Susan's parents. First, given her role in court proceedings, it was necessary for her to form an independent opinion of the parents' relationships with their children and their potential for change. It was important for the children therapeutically and probably for the parents that the therapist acknowledged them as the children's natural parents, and therefore as playing a pivotal role in their children's lives. It is also helpful for the therapist when working with children to have first-hand experience of their parents, including their appearance, tones of voice, unique phrases, posture and gait, and more general personality characteristics. Given this direct contact, the therapist can then recognise more readily in therapy sessions when the child is referring to a parent, or is perhaps adopting a parental role or instructing the therapist to do so, or when the child unconsciously imitates a parent's characteristics.

Introductory meetings with the child

While there can be circumstances in which a therapist meets a child for the first time in the play therapy room, in most cases it is advisable to meet the child at home or in another familiar environment first. One of the primary tasks of the therapist is to create for the child as quickly as possible an atmosphere in the playroom of permissiveness and security. This permissiveness will enable a troubled child to relax and begin to explore emotionally difficult areas of experience. Children seem less threatened by the unfamiliarity of the play therapy room if the therapist is not a complete stranger to them.

At their first meeting the therapist is conveying by her actions, words and responses her general manner and attitudes towards children. For example, in her visit with Susan and her brothers, the therapist tried to demonstrate her attitudes of friendliness and non-intrusiveness, as well as an orientation of giving primary attention to the children themselves, rather than, say, spending most of the visit talking with Cath about her concerns. She also tried to respond immediately and appropriately to each of the children's interactions – or lack of them – with her.

Inexperienced therapists sometimes treat an introductory visit as a preliminary piece of work in which principles of play therapy need not apply. However, this visit, like any interaction with the child, is an important one and the child's initial reaction to the therapist gives information in itself about the child. With Susan and her brothers the visit also provided first-hand information on the children's interactions with one another and with Cath. An additional advantage of a home visit is that the therapist can observe the behaviour of the child in a setting other than the playroom. She will then be able to have a basis for comparison with the child's reactions during sessions. The visit will strengthen or call into question many hypotheses the therapist has formulated at referral. It will also generate new questions, as our chapter on assessment will illustrate in more detail.

In the introductory visit, the therapist was careful to introduce herself immediately, and explained what her job was, who had referred the children and what the general problem was for which they had been referred. She stated this problem in general terms in order to leave room open to the children to interpret this in their own way. Too much information about the children's lives at this point and too much specification of their problem would have been overly directive and also too threatening to them, judging from their already anxious reactions to her visit. She changed the topic to a more enjoyable one, the playroom, rather than continuing with more information about their parents at the beginning, looking for an opportunity to refer to them at some more appropriate point later in the visit.

For these reasons it is important, therefore, to keep the pace of the visit slow and relaxed enough for the child to have time, if s/he wishes, to think about what is said and ask any questions. It is also crucial that the therapist's attitude be one of attentiveness and alertness to the child's verbal and non-verbal responses. The child's behaviour and verbalisations should determine the timing and detail of the information the therapist gives. The therapist will throughout the visit be practising the key therapeutic skill of recognising and reflecting the child's feelings. However, in beginning work some of the child's feelings may be recognised by the therapist, but legitimately judged to be too inhibiting and intrusive or too threatening to the child for the therapist to acknowledge overtly. An example from the visit with Susan and her brothers would be Gerry's avoidance of any direct eye contact and Susan's overactivity. The therapist needs to have developed an ability to engage in heightened observation of the child (Wilson, 1992) as well as a sensitivity to the timing and contents of his or her remarks.

In introducing information to the child which will be needed to understand the purpose of play therapy, information that the therapist suspects will be highly emotive for a child is best conveyed in the presence of a supportive carer, and after the child's initial anxiety about meeting the therapist has diminished somewhat. With Susan and her brothers the therapist waited to talk about her letter to their parents, the court process and the limits to confidentiality with them until towards the end of her visit. She decided to do this in Cath's presence, rather than discussing these topics immediately or waiting until their first play therapy session together. She was also acknowledging to the children that their parents still remained their parents, even though their foster carers had made strong commitments to the children. Their parents were potentially still important emotionally to the children and still had a right to information about important events in their lives.

She was also trying to acknowledge that their carers and social worker had roles of their own in the children's lives which she as therapist would not replace. Children who are looked after, as mentioned above, often have to form relationships with adult professionals which are unlike those of other children their age. With Susan and her brothers it is evident that issues such as the ones mentioned above are not just emotionally but intellectually complicated for a child. Often the child needs time and more than one opportunity to process this kind of information. The issue of confidentiality was raised, for example, in the introductory visit and was returned to by Susan in her first session as one that was difficult but important to her in her own particular way. When such an issue is raised in the presence of the carer (and to a lesser extent, in the presence of the siblings), a child will be able to go over the topic in a general way with the carer and other family members after the introductory visit. Most carers would be experienced in helping a child process a new and anxiety-provoking experience, but with some carers the therapist may have explicitly to mention that the children will need the carer's help in understanding what the therapist said in her visit.

Practice issues in the first session

In our first book we discussed some of the practice issues with a child beginning therapy, such as the child's initial fearfulness and the therapist's need to establish trust by showing sensitivity to the child's often largely non-verbal responses. Another practice issue will be featured here which centres on the therapist herself: the therapist's attitude of 'free-floating attentiveness' and the internal mental focus the therapist must maintain during her first session with a child.

The therapist's primary focus must, as we have said, be on the child in the first session; her own feelings and reactions in relation to the child, however, also need to be processed in relation to the child she is encountering. As we have discussed it was difficult for the therapist to detect Susan's reaction of distress when paint went into her eye. She was able quickly to recognize that Susan was in discomfort by her knowledge that children from abusive environments sometimes suffer discomfort or pain silently, rather than attracting possible indifferent or hostile reaction from their carers. But she herself also experienced internal guilt at not having prevented Susan's distress. She was aware of reacting with more guilt in the therapy session than in an ordinary play situation not only because of a personal tendency to magnify guilty responses, but also because therapy is by definition intended to be a very safe, supportive environment. Yet in this instance it had been a source of distress for Susan. She felt a need to protect Susan from further emotional and/or physical distress because she had already experienced a repeatedly abusive environment. Susan's reaction of passivity and heightened dependence brought out this feeling strongly – a response which would be more appropriate normally to have with a baby or toddler than with a six-year-old girl. In other words, even in this brief interaction, the therapist was monitoring her responses for her personal reactions, which would give her clues to understanding Susan's personality and experiences.

Another personal and somewhat negative reaction to Susan was the feeling of dismay at the mess she would have to clean up after the session. From experience of working with children who needed to express their inner turmoil by outward disorder, the therapist was already convinced that this behaviour was important for children. She therefore accepted its aftermath more easily and was also confident of being able to set limits to Susan's messiness, if they were needed. But given Susan's fear of adverse adult reactions, limit-setting would have to be done without any trace of adult disapproval or negativity, otherwise her tendency to explore the environment would probably be curtailed.

Within this context it is important for the therapist to be aware of the limits to her personal tolerance. When the therapist is very concerned that she cannot keep a child under control or if she herself cannot tolerate a particular behaviour, these 'emotive messages' will usually be picked up by the child. The child will often respond by becoming more anxious about boundaries, either escalating 'bad' behaviour to ensure strong reaction from the adult or, as Susan might have done, restricting spontaneous behaviour and feelings.

To facilitate self-awareness and awareness of the child's ongoing thoughts and feelings, before beginning a session the therapist needs to attempt to attain a particular kind of conscious state. Freud advocated a state of 'free-floating' attention to the contents of clients' associations; Reik in turn labelled this stance 'listening with the third ear' (Bettelheim and Rosenfeld, 1993). The necessary freeing of the therapist's mind from everyday concerns has also been seen as akin to the 'emptying' of the mind practised in meditation and Zen Bhuddism. The therapist's state of mind, then, needs to be one in which personal or outside agendas are put aside, by being digested or held in store. At the same time she must adopt an attitude of general attentiveness to the child with specific attentiveness and processing of the child's words and actions. This generalised attentiveness to the child is emphasised and clarified in non-directive play therapy by reflective listening, as we discuss in the next section.

The therapist in practice needs to make specific provision for herself to achieve this state of 'free-floating attention' to the child. An effective way to achieve this is for the therapist deliberately to schedule a short preparation time before the therapy hour, and use this time to prepare both the room for the child and to prepare herself internally for being receptive to the child's state of mind. Before the first session, as we detailed in our earlier book, the therapist will need time to think carefully about the child's age and circumstances and to decide on the appropriate play materials and arrangement of the room for this particular child, since the room will remain the same each subsequent week. Emotional and intellectual commitments which are too demanding in other areas of the therapist's work, or a preoccupation with serious personal problems will make achieving this state of mind extremely difficult, especially for an inexperienced therapist.

The therapist's ability to view the child as a new and unique person is vital to the establishment of their relationship in the first session, and remains a feature of the therapeutic relationship with the child even after many sessions. Sometimes it is difficult for an experienced therapist to view the child in this fresh way when she has worked with many children with similar histories. At other times it is more difficult because of the therapist's heightened anxiety about beginning this work, perhaps because of a consciousness of her own inadequacy or inexperience, and other times because the child's problems seem so intractible.

The therapist's openness to the child is also essential to the development of a genuine therapeutic relationship. This new relationship with the child is: '. . . a mutual journey of discovery. And at least about the topic of who he is and why he does what he does, [the child] is as much of an authority as you and possesses far more pertinent facts. He will sense your alertness, curiosity and humility and will respond to these, often in a positive fashion' (Bettelheim and Rosenfeld, 1993: 29).

These authors go on to discuss the necessity of having curiosity about the therapeutic relationship with a child, in order for the therapist herself to have an intellectual and emotional investment in the process. This curiosity in our experience is necessary not only to offset any reaction of 'sameness' and boredom to the everyday occurrences in play therapy with children, but also to offset the initial anxiety the therapist feels in any new encounter with a child.

From the child's viewpoint the therapist's curiosity is vital as well. Children need to have their sense of self developed within relationships with significant others (see Wilson et al., 1992, Chapter 7). Their need to make themselves understood works in tandem with their activity of explaining and experiencing themselves in new ways in relation to the therapist. If, as Bettelheim and Rosenfeld point out, the therapist always reacts to the child's new insights and behaviours with a lack of surprise and interest, the child might ask why he or she should bother to continue with self-exploration and internal changes, if the therapist knows everything already!

As we discuss elsewhere, the therapeutic situation mimics a child–carer relationship in important respects (Ryan and Wilson, 1995a), with the parent normally responding to the child's new-found knowledge and ability with pleasure and excitement over the child's development. The therapist's attitudes of general attentiveness and of curiosity are, we think, easier to maintain in non-directive play therapy compared to more directive approaches. The first session with Susan demonstrates the ways in which this encounter was unique and unplanned by the therapist. The therapist, especially before the first session, then, needs a curiosity about the child she will meet and a general sense of attentiveness in the first session to the child's unique personality. And, as we illustrate next with Patrick, and then throughout the book, not only are children's personalities varied and inherently interesting, but their situations and requirements can change substantially during the course of their play therapy sessions.

Chapter 2

Patrick
From Concrete to Symbolic Play

*Many arrivals make us live: the tree becoming
Green, a bird tipping the topmost bough,
A seed pushing itself beyond itself,...*
  Theodore Roethke,'The Manifestation'

The play therapy sessions described in this chapter concern Patrick, a four-year-old boy who had been sexually abused and emotionally neglected by his young parents before he was taken into care. Play therapy was offered to help him redress these psychologically damaging early experiences. We shall first describe Patrick himself, his background, current life and the future plans being made for him by the local authority. We then give an account of his therapeutic play sessions, which clearly illustrate the ways a child can move from very concrete, circumscribed play to develop the more normal capacity to play on a symbolic level. The discussion which follows explores the practice issues which arose for the therapist. These include the demanding task of responding appropriately to a child with rudimentary language development, the necessity for a high level of consistency in the therapist's responses and the role of the therapist when allegations of abuse are made by the child during ongoing play therapy sessions. Although we do not explore this practice issue in detail here, it will again be apparent, as it has been in the first chapter and throughout this book, that the child's total environment is crucial in effecting general and longlasting changes in his psychological functioning.

In the final section we explore some of the theoretical implications of Patrick's sessions, examining the notion of play therapy as an artificially enhanced environment, and demonstrating some ways in which an awareness of normal development is necessary both to increase our understanding of therapeutic responses to a child and in assessing a child's therapeutic progress. We conclude by considering the role of symbolisation in play therapy and in normal development.

PATRICK'S BACKGROUND

Patrick was almost four years old when he was removed from his parents and placed in his current foster home, where he had been for four months when our sessions started. His foster carers were a late middle-aged couple, Louise and Steve, whose own three children were now young adults. Patrick's parents were themselves in their early twenties and Patrick was their first child. His father and mother had lived together for several years in council estate housing and were cut off from their own family ties. Neither of them had been able to find employment, nor did they seem to have any marketable educational or vocational skills. Their main interest appeared to be their wide group of 'mates', and their music and video collection. Patrick's parents had come to the attention of social services because of an allegation that his father had sexually abused a six-year-old child. There had been an investigation and his father had been convicted of indecent exposure and had been imprisoned for six months. This had been his first offence and he had explained his actions to the court as 'totally unusual' and 'due to the stress of being out of work'. Patrick's mother had continued during this time to care for Patrick by herself and her care of him had been monitored by the local authority. Although Patrick's social worker had minor concerns over his timidity and lack of communication, as well as his somewhat slow development, she judged that these difficulties resulted from impoverishment and suspicion of her statutory role. His mother appeared to be providing adequately for Patrick's physical care and to be protecting him from any potentially abusive situations.

Patrick had regular contact with his father, being taken by his mother on her fortnightly visits to his father in prison. When the social worker talked with Patrick's mother about the difficult child protection issues surrounding his father returning to live with them after his release from prison, she had been noncommital concerning her future relationship with him. She stated that 'she'd have to see', while refusing any counselling or assessment herself on her future ability to protect Patrick. Both parents were told that his father would need to undergo an assessment and treatment programme for sex offenders before a decision could be made by the local authority about his returning to live with his family.

They had also been warned that if he returned before these assessments, Patrick would need to live away from his mother because of doubts about her ability to protect Patrick adequately from his father's possible abuse of him.

Despite these warnings, Patrick's father in fact immediately resumed his relationship with his family on his release from prison. As a result of this, four months before Patrick's referral to me, he had been removed from his mother's care.

It was only after Patrick came into care that his social worker and foster carers began to suspect that Patrick had been subjected to emotional abuse and traumatisation or neglect by his parents. After a period of extreme passivity and watchfulness in his first weeks at his foster home, Patrick began to relax more and to join in the family's activities. They increasingly noticed that, although Patrick was quick to learn, he appeared to have delayed language and motor skills and an inability to play. Patrick also began to talk to Louise and Steve in very unclear language, with many accompanying gestures, about incidents involving his father and mother which sounded sexually abusive. Louise kept a diary of events from the beginning of his placement, recording these and other worrying behaviour by Patrick, along with his general adjustment and important events for him while in their care.

Louise had noted in her diary that Patrick from the beginning had generally remained passive and without emotion, but had become very agitated at any mention of the toilet and had refused to go himself or be taken there. They had compromised by allowing him to use a child's potty outside the door to the toilet for the time being. As Patrick settled into his placement with them Louise talked to him about starting to use the toilet. Patrick became very agitated once more and began to talk about his parents hurting him and then, holding his genital and anal areas, excitedly pointed to the toilet. Patrick had remained silent when Louise explained to him that they needed to go and talk to someone else about what Patrick was telling her.

After giving me the above information at our referral meeting, Cathy, Patrick's social worker, said how dismayed she'd been by the investigative interview. It 'had been a waste of time' evidentially, since Patrick seemed unable to talk to her about himself as he did with Louise. In fact, she thought it had impaired her relationship with him, because Patrick was more withdrawn in her company now. Patrick's subsequent medical examination confirmed slight anal scarring, which could possibly have been due to adult sexual abuse, but was not definitive.

When Cathy and I met with Louise before Patrick's sessions began, Louise confirmed that Patrick's great agitation surrounding the toilet was in strong contrast to his usual emotional responses, which were flat and unspontaneous. She had never seen Patrick angry in the four months he had lived with them. He was more talkative now, but he continually asked her permission, or her husband's when she wasn't nearby, before he did anything. Cathy confirmed this behaviour, saying that Patrick was also very quiet in his weekly access visits with his mother, which they had just begun to supervise following Patrick's allegations, since these seemed to be against both his parents. (Patrick's father had refused to attend any contact visits since Patrick had been removed from home, saying he objected to 'being spied on by a bloody social worker'.) Cathy added that Patrick was easily overlooked by his mother during their contact time together because she often spent much of her time talking with the social worker who was supervising their visits about her grievances against the department and concerns over Patrick's care. She made few attempts to engage Patrick in play and conversation, even though the supervisor continually tried to bring his mother's attention back to him.

Patrick was attending a playgroup on three mornings a week and the playgroup leader had described Patrick as very withdrawn and quiet; he was also unable readily to play with the other children. She had found that he liked one-to-one attention by an adult, especially on construction activities and puzzles. Patrick seemed to concentrate well during this kind of activity and had rapidly learned in his two months with them to use new implements and materials.

We then discussed in general terms the court report Cathy had asked me to write for the pending care proceedings with Patrick, in addition to my therapeutic work with him. I described the method, aims and potential effects of non-directive play therapy and the professional support arrangements for the foster carers. I also emphasised, as we arranged the practical details of time, place and transport, the importance of regular, predictable sessions for Patrick.

In my introductory meeting with him in his foster home, Patrick seemed for the most part to be withdrawn and not to want either Louise or me to notice him. We had a cup of tea together and Louise and I talked more generally with Patrick taking small glances at me from the other side of the room from time to time. After a while, first glancing at Patrick briefly and changing my voice tone, I addressed Louise, saying that she knew about Patrick coming lots of times, and that she would bring him to talk and play with me. I added that I would try to help him with anything that worried him. I also left photos of the building and playroom with Louise, with a comment that she could show Patrick later if he wanted to see them. They could give them back to me when they came to the playroom. Patrick walked to the door with Louise and held her hand as I left, looking solemn and watchful.

I also met with Patrick's parents, who listened to a brief explanation of my method of working with Patrick, but were unable or perhaps unwilling to describe Patrick to me when I asked them about their view of him. Neither of them could remember more than the most rudimentary details of Patrick's early life with them, even when we went step by step over Patrick's pre-birth and birth, his infancy and early childhood. It was difficult to engage them in conversation and even more difficult to help them keep their focus on Patrick during the first part of the hour's interview. Once we began to discuss what Patrick needed, they both became more animated and began to berate me for not taking the side of Patrick's father, who still maintained his innocence, despite his conviction. They continued by blaming the local authority for removing their son without any 'good reason', with Patrick's mother protesting that she had always looked after Patrick properly, and his father arguing that he was still being punished for something he hadn't done by Patrick being taken away. I attempted to focus on what Patrick needed from his parents, now that he was being looked after by the local authority, but they were unable to respond positively, saying that they 'loved him and wanted him back; that's what he needs'. We ended by my offering to meet with them again if they had questions or comments on Patrick's play therapy that Cathy was unable to help them with.

PATRICK'S PLAY THERAPY SESSIONS

Patrick's first response in the playroom surprised me. I had expected that his withdrawal from me at his foster carers' would be even more pronounced in the new environment of the playroom. Instead, he came upstairs holding Louise's hand and looking interested in where he was being taken. (I made a mental note to tell Cathy when I had the opportunity how well they seemed to have prepared Patrick for this experience.) I showed them both where drinks could be made in the kitchen and where Louise would be waiting for Patrick to finish. I then showed them where the toilet was, and said to Patrick that there was a potty there too and that Louise had mentioned to me he might want it. I also reassured Patrick that he could go to Louise if he needed her help when he wanted to use the toilet, or that he could let me help him or do it himself.

Before entering the playroom, we all went into the video equipment room and I talked with them about being on TV when we were in the playroom. Patrick turned and asked Louise if he could push the button. Louise explained to me that Patrick was allowed to do this at home when she or Steve were there and I agreed that, after I put the video in, Patrick could press the button. After he did this and waited at the screen, I explained to him that I would look at it later to remember what we did together, and showed him that it wasn't like his tapes at home. I'd be the only one to look at it and write about it. I would tell him first if anybody else needed to see it. Then I told him that I'd lock the room with my key and we'd go to the playroom. Patrick's manner throughout this introduction seemed contented. Although I wasn't certain he had understood or even listened to all the information I had given him, I intended to repeat this routine with some of the accompanying information where appropriate at the beginning of our next sessions.

Patrick had taken Louise's hand again on the way to the playroom, but released his hold as soon as he entered. He moved directly over to the sand tray near the door, looking over the sand toys very intently and at length. I explained to Patrick that he could play with whatever he wanted when he came to this room. All the things were there for him to use. Louise said goodbye to him saying she'd be in the waiting room all the time. Patrick said goodbye, glancing up briefly, and then remained looking at the sand. He hesitantly touched the toy spade sticking out of the sand, while I talked about his not being sure about the sand, but that it did look good to him, too. I noticed how he glanced at me before each small action he performed: glancing before getting the spade out of the sand and again before digging with it gently on the surface of the sand. I responded by saying that Patrick wanted to be sure it was all right to do it and again reassuring him that he could play with all the things in the room.

When Patrick looked at the sand and then at me, I smiled and looked at him briefly, adopting a quiet, waiting posture. He then began to dig more systematically, filling all the containers on the surface of the sand tray with great concentration. I remained silent for most of this activity, only commenting briefly about how busy Patrick was and how he wanted to fill them to the very top with sand. (I wanted to talk a little in order to keep contact with him and to demonstrate my – hopefully! – benign presence in his play activity.) I was interested that Patrick seemed to avoid handling any toys that had sand sticking to them, even though the sand was dry, while he filled the containers. I remarked, 'You don't like that one', as he lightly touched the edge of a sandy bucket and immediately withdrew his hand, 'Maybe it's too messy for you'.

For about 15 minutes Patrick filled the containers, until all the clean ones visible to him had been filled. Then he looked up from the sand box and towards me, then looked at the shelf near us, letting his glance remain on the middle shelf. I again responded that he had seen something and might want to find out what it was, repeating once again that the toys were there for him to play with. Patrick remained rigidly in his same position at the sand tray, looking towards the shelf. I offered to get what he was looking at, saying maybe he wanted me to help him. Patrick nodded and I got the game down on which he had seemed to focus. It had a hammer and individual plastic circles with counters on them to hit down repeatedly as they randomly popped up. He immediately began to set the counters himself and I commented that he seemed to know how to work them himself.

After setting the counters Patrick tapped the hammer gently on the circles but did not depress the raised areas. (The game is based on vigorous hitting and quick reflexes, and usually played in a loud, banging fashion.) He then hesitated before slowly squeezing the raised areas with both hands in order to depress them slightly. I commented that maybe Patrick knew how to play the game but didn't want to hit them hard. Maybe he wondered if it would be too noisy here. I told him clearly that children could be noisy in the playroom with me and that lots of children liked to be noisy when they played that game. Patrick spent some minutes squeezing the pieces in the game, then turned to examine the lid to the box, which had a photograph of the game's contents and two children looking at them, their mouths open in surprised delight. Patrick became engrossed in matching the real items to the items shown on the lid and then began to study the photograph of the boy and girl intently. After a pause he pointed to the children, saying, 'Crying'. I replied, 'Maybe not crying. Maybe happy and surprised'. (Slight pause) 'But you think they're crying'. Patrick stared intently at the boy, repeating 'Crying', softly to himself. He then returned to the sand for the remainder of the hour, emptying and filling the containers, being careful to pour them out and fill them without allowing the sand to touch his hands, as I resumed my role of quietly commenting on what he was doing from close by the sand tray.

Patrick quickly developed a routine in his sessions. I deliberately began them in the same way each time Louise brought him upstairs. We viewed the kitchen and toilet, went into the video room and Patrick pushed the 'record' button. I then locked the door after us and Louise came with us into the playroom. Patrick would immediately go to the sand tray from our second session onwards and say goodbye to Louise from there. He slowly began to become more spontaneous in his exploration of the room, in his interactions with me, and with the materials and toys he allowed himself to use in the room. From playing exclusively with the containers, Patrick began to indicate to me that I should pull out the sandy toys and brush them off for him to use, looking intently at me while I performed this action. I talked about my liking the sand and not minding when it went on my hands. I could brush the sand off again. (I demonstrated this action sometimes to Patrick as he watched me closely.) 'But you don't like the sand on your hands. You want me to do it for you.'

I also commented on how he wanted to play in the sand, but it was hard for him to do, as Patrick began sometimes to pull the edge of a toy out of the sand with his fingertips.

During one of his early sessions Patrick as usual began his hour by filling containers with sand at the sand tray, telling me to get the sandy toys stuck out in the sand out for him.

> V: [complying with his request] I can help you. I like to put my hands in the sand. You don't like it.
> P: [staring at my hands] Wash them *now*.
> V: I will go and wash them for you, but I could just brush it off like this [showing him how].
> P: Wash them.
> V: Yes. You need me to wash them.

Patrick repeated similar sequences of diffident, yet persistent actions with other materials in the playroom. With the playdough, he motioned me to reach in to take the cool, slightly sticky, damp-feeling playdough out of its container, after struggling unsuccessfully for some time to remove it himself using a spoon. As I touched the playdough myself with my fingers while he watched, Patrick looked very upset, seeming to be simultaneously repelled and attracted to this clinging, messy substance. He also began to use the paints, first in a very circumscribed way and appearing very fearful that his hands would be contaminated. He progressed to becoming engrossed in covering a paper solidly with paint after indicating to me that I too should paint next to him, watching before he started that I did so. He began to order me to follow his lead, dipping my brush into the colour he chose for me and motioning me to copy his painting. (We discuss this dynamic of pseudo-autonomy in the case study of Helen, in chapter 4 of our earlier book). But each time he accidentally got a spot of paint on his hands, Patrick rushed over to the basin and washed them thoroughly. He watched with surprise as I got a bit of paint on my hands and did not appear to mind. I commented, 'Painting is very messy to do, and it's fun too'. But Patrick became distressed and ordered me to wash my hands. Complying, I commented that it wasn't fun for him if we got too messy; that upset him. As I washed my hands, I said 'I wasn't bothered. I can wait until I finish. But I can wash them now if that makes you feel better'.

After washing his hands during his painting activity a few times, Patrick left the painting and began to experiment with the drinking containers on the side of the basin. Using the feeder cup, baby's bottle, cup and small pitcher containing orange juice Patrick started to pour juice back and forth among the containers, with a laugh erupting intermittently from him as he played. I joined in his laughter when he looked towards me, and Patrick began to giggle and take sips from the cup and feeder cup, turning slightly away from me again. With disapproval in his voice, he told me that the bottle was for a baby. I replied that it was, but sometimes children liked to play with it too. This bottle was for children to play with; babies were too little to come to the playroom with me. Patrick looked again at the bottle, then abruptly put the containers down and went to the soft sponge ball. Smiling to himself, he gently kicked the ball from place to place in the room. Then he returned abruptly to the drink containers, seeming to be deliberately avoiding looking at the bottle. He sipped the orange drink, filled the cup to the brim again, sipped, poured it out, and refilled it to the brim, smiling as he played. Afterwards he turned to the baby bottle, looked directly at it and managed to pick it up very hesitantly.

Fiddling with the top for a while, engrossed, Patrick turned to ask me for help in unscrewing it, then asked me if I wanted a drink, repeating that he was too big:

V: I don't mind. If you want me to.

Patrick got me to screw the top back on after he had filled the bottle with orange drink by himself.

P: You drink it.
V: All right. Maybe I'm a baby?
P: Yeah.
V: Waah! Where's my bottle?

He smiled slightly and gave me the bottle to drink. I drank it, making satisfied noises ['Mmmmm'] as I did so. Patrick watched very intently, but without any signs of enjoyment at my pretend play. I finished sucking the bottle after a short time.

V: [smiling] It's very odd to see a big lady drinking a bottle.

I drank a bit more while Patrick stared intently.

P: Want some more?
V: I can. I don't really drink out of a bottle, do I? I'm just playing I'm drinking out of a bottle now.

Patrick then started pretending, although very unsurely, that he was taking the carer's role, telling me to wait while he refilled the bottle, and managing to unscrew and screw it again himself. He gave me more to drink.

P: Drink it.
V: [smiling] You're taking care of me, giving me lots of drinks.

I drank, then paused to laugh while briefly glancing directly at Patrick, who smiled slightly. (This sequence is also discussed in Ryan and Wilson, 1995a: 35.)

After this, in his next sessions Patrick continued his play with water, paints, playdough and sand and his interactions with me became more relaxed and spontaneous. He began to have periods of kicking the soft ball to me with evident enjoyment and we laughed together happily. Then he began to throw the ball to me, and his laughter became louder, especially when I missed catching some of his wilder shots. He continued too to wash his hands often, starting to put the plug into the basin and half-filling the basin with water in the process. After enjoying the sensation of the running water on his hands, Patrick ended up plunging both his hands into the water up to his elbows, wriggling his fingers while they remained under the water and laughing with pleasure. He then had me put my hands in the water with him and after enjoying the experience together, Patrick had us play at tickling one another's fingers.

Patrick also branched out to other play activities. He played with the figures in the doll's house, naming himself along with members of his foster family as he put them through their routine daily activities, such as going upstairs, watching TV and getting into bed. The figure representing himself became more prominent in his play as the sessions went on. Patrick familiarised himself with the house's rooms and furniture, and then placed the doll near the room in the house with the play toilet and bath. He told me he didn't like the big toilet.

V: You're a big boy now, but you don't like the big toilet.
P: Louise lets me.
V: You're pleased Louise lets you [use the potty].
P: Big toilet's bad!
V: You think it's very bad for you, the big toilet.
P: [in anguished tone] Mummy, Daddy [holding genitals] hurt there.
V: They hurt you? You're holding yourself there [looking at Patrick's hands].
P: Hurt wee-wee. Mummy, Daddy did!
V: Your Mummy and Daddy hurt your wee-wee.
P: Big toilet bad! [throwing it out of the doll's house]
V: You want to throw the big toilet away! Your mummy and daddy hurt you. You don't want to be hurt any more.

Patrick nodded fiercely and kicked the toilet further away from us.

V: I don't want you to be hurt any more either. I need to tell Cathy about it. About your telling me that your mummy and daddy hurt your wee-wee near the toilet.

Patrick nodded and returned to the doll, placing it in the bath and pretending to bathe it gently, then got it out and readied it for bed.

V: He's liking that. He likes you to be soft and gentle [adopting a soft tone of voice].

Patrick continued to play easily and went back to Louise in a relaxed, chatty mood at the end of the session.

Patrick began to spend part of his sessions cutting with scissors out of the box of drawing materials on the table. He struggled himself for a time, engrossed in controlling the scissors with two hands and trying to prevent the paper from slipping out from between the scissor's blades. I quietly offered to hold the paper, if he needed me to help him, but Patrick did not respond at all to my suggestion. He continued to struggle with the effort of cutting the paper himself, managed to cut into the paper from the edge several times, then put it aside and went to the other side of the room and began to climb cautiously onto the round, soft, two-foot high play cushion there. First he placed his tummy on the cushion, looking at me, and I gave my reassurance that it was there for children to play on. Patrick then allowed himself to wriggle forward and lift his legs up onto the cushion, reaching out his hand for me to help him.

During his next sessions he allowed me to hold the paper for him as he practised cutting for extended periods of time. I occasionally reflected his feelings about wanting to do it better, of his doing it more easily when I helped him hold the paper and how it was hard to do. He was intent on the task of cutting and did not respond, nor did I require a response from him, making certain that my comments would not distract him from concentrating on an activity which seemed so important to him to practise.

Following one lengthy period of cutting Patrick began to notice and pick up the pieces he had cut, walked over and put them behind a chair, saying they were for 'the lady crying'. I reflected Patrick's feelings of wanting to be kind to the lady, to help her. When Patrick repeated his play sequence several times with a serious look on his face, I commented that maybe it upset him to see her crying, maybe she was crying a lot. He at last seemed satisfied and I reflected this feeling, as well as Patrick's shift to another less intense activity. (But I was aware with all my comments that I did not know what associations Patrick had to 'the lady crying' or why this enactment was emotionally so important to him. I could simply help him by talking about the nature and strength of his feelings. I later checked with both Cathy and Louise, as well as the guardian and court papers, but I could not directly relate this to a past experience in Patrick's life.)

Before our fifteenth session I was told by Cathy that Louise would be going into hospital for several days for a scheduled operation. Patrick would be told by Louise and Steve that Louise would be gone for a few days, and that Steve would be caring for him while she was away. They seemed to feel it was important to protect Patrick from the real reason for Louise's absence, since he had been through so much and was becoming devoted to her. I replied that he needed to know that Louise would go to the hospital and that a straightforward reason should be given (perhaps 'because the doctor needed to help her so she didn't get so many tummyaches any more'). Any subsequent questions of his also needed to be answered in a simple, reassuring and direct way. We also talked about possible strategies for helping Patrick wait for Louise's return, such as identifying an object which was immediately recognisable as being exclusively Louise's which she used regularly, and entrusting Patrick to 'take care of it' for her until she came home. Telephone calls from Louise at least daily, especially if Patrick was unable to visit her in the hospital, would also be important to him.

Patrick arrived for our fifteenth session holding on to Steve's hand tightly, with a child-sized bag in his other hand. After Steve said goodbye to him at the door to the playroom, Patrick put his bag down and started running round the room haphazardly, with what looked like nervous energy. He climbed on to the soft play cushion (he was now quite adept at this activity), jumped off several times and insisted that I allow him to climb on to the table by the window.

> V: I'll pull this chair up to the window and I'll stay near you, but you can't be on the table. You might get hurt there.
> V: [as I moved the chair and Patrick tugged at his hair] You're upset today, Patrick.
> P: [after climbing on to the chair and beginning to scrape his fingernails on the window] I'm bashing now!
> V: No, no bashing. The window might break and then the glass can cut you.

Patrick raised his fist and I held his arm.

> V: [firmly] No bashing. I have to take care of you. I don't want you to get hurt.

Patrick relaxed his arm and stood leaning into me on the chair. We talked about everything he could see and hear from the window – the man walking the dog on the pavement, the car going by, the climbing frame in the garden . . . and I remembered the many times I had been with my own children as toddlers, just like this, looking out of a window while holding them in a loose embrace and both of us giving our attention to absorbing the minutiae of the world passing by.

Patrick eventually picked up a pen top and, having tried to insert it into the window lock a few times, decided to get down. He went to his own bag, looked at it, said that the play cushion was a bag, then started rolling the cushion on its side towards me, looking at me easily and laughing. I talked about the bag coming to me and the bag going back to him. He evolved this motion into a play sequence in which the life-sized play telephone booth in the corner of the playroom was the house. We squeezed in there together (a tight fit – I was grateful I didn't weigh a stone or two more!) and I commented on how we were close together in the house. Patrick sat next to me, smiling up at me, then took his bag and said goodbye to me. I talked about Patrick going off and leaving me by myself in the house, while he crawled under the table and lay down. He remained very quiet, and I said that I couldn't see and hear him. I was all by myself. I wondered where he was. I asked Patrick if maybe I wanted to see him but I couldn't. Patrick nodded vehemently and said 'You cry'. (Note how much surer and more complete my reflections of Patrick's feelings here were compared with those about 'the lady crying' earlier.)

I cried, saying I wanted him and didn't want to be on my own in the house. Patrick then had me roll the cushion back and forth across the room with him again and again, getting more excited as we continued. He told me to go back into the 'house' and he returned with his bag in hand, squeezing in beside me and smiling up at me. I reflected that I felt so good that he was with me again. And that Patrick was happy to be home with me, too. Patrick repeated this play sequence twice more during the session, giving me instructions as we carried out the actions that I should bring some toys into my house and start playing while he was gone. I was then able to talk about how I could play at home and I knew he'd come back to be with me in the house soon. Patrick seem satisfied with this response, got his bag and, for the first time, decided to leave our session early. I commented to him that he'd finished for today and played what he wanted to play. Now he needed to find Steve.

Steve brought Patrick for the next two sessions. During these sessions Patrick's manner was more intense and also more active than when he had come with Louise. He again played through the play sequence with the 'house' and bag from the week before but began to play out activities in which he was the carer looking after the child (me). I was given a bath, sitting in the large dressing up clothes box, it having been emptied by Patrick for us to use (with me having a quick inner smile about how daft I'd later appear on the video). I was also made to look smart, getting my best clothes on and my hair brushed. Patrick wanted me to take off my shoes and put on another pair. He watched as I removed my shoes, but became very fearful when he saw my toes (since it was high summer I had bare feet). I immediately went to put my shoes back on, saying that he looked frightened of my toes. Patrick sighed heavily and I told him that now he felt better. He was very frightened when he saw my toes, but I wouldn't hurt him. Patrick listened, looked again at my shoes and smiled up at me. He then went over to the paints and we painted together, with Patrick directing my actions but allowing both of us to continue painting, even when we accidentally got paint on our fingers.

At the beginning of our next session Patrick climbed the stairs with his face wreathed in smiles, holding triumphantly on to Louise's hand.

V: You're *so pleased*. Louise's here again, Patrick!
P: Look at the sand, Louise! [plunging his hand in and showing her a handful] Look at the house! No banging on the window, Louise. She can be my baby in here! [talking quickly and excitedly pulling Louise around the room]
V: You want to show Louise everything! You missed Louise a lot. Now she's here with you again!

He spent several minutes with Louise before she left to wait nearby.

At the end of our eighteenth session, I told Patrick that we had two more times together, in order to allow him enough time to think about the end of our time together. In my final progress meeting with Cathy and Louise, which also occurred about this time, we exchanged information on Patrick's progress. We all felt that he had benefited greatly from his play therapy sessions. His playgroup had reported that Patrick was starting to play with other children, but still remained somewhat on the periphery of any group. Both the playgroup and Louise had noticed that Patrick was learning many new skills very quickly now, and everyone who knew him had commented on how much more spontaneous and exhuberant he had become recently, and very much more able to laugh and race happily around. His speech was also developing rapidly; he was able to understand more complex sentences and he was beginning to enjoy basic jokes and to volunteer to sing nursery rhymes to Louise and Steve's relatives when they came to the house.

Patrick spent our last two sessions playing with most of the toys in the room and engaging me in carer–child play sequences. These sequences were interspersed with having me sit at the far end of the room, where I was able to comment that Patrick was putting me far away from him, and seeing what it was like to play on his own.

I heard about Patrick's progress from time to time in the next several years after our sessions together and after my court involvement in his case had ended. He went to live with his adoptive parents who were very sensitive to his sadness and anger at his departure from Louise and Steve, and were able to accept his increased fearfulness and clinging behaviour to them. (The decision to move him and to place him in a new adoptive home, given his attachment to Louise and Steve, had not been easy, but in the end both foster carers and the social workers felt that he would be better placed with younger adoptive parents, and that he would be able to form close attachments to them, as indeed proved the case.) His new parents did need additional psychological consultations about a year after Patrick went to live with them to help them with some of Patrick's persistent problems related to fearfulness. They also intend to continue their contact with the psychologist in order to have ready access to consultations and monitoring of Patrick's developmental progress for the future. In addition, the social work support during the adoption process and for an extended period of time afterwards seemed beneficial to Patrick and his new family.

PRACTICE ISSUES

Communicating with young children

Patrick's sessions show that there are certain communication skills which the therapist needs to develop in order to work with a young child who has had both restricted and damaging early learning experiences. (See, for example, Mogford-Bevan, 1994, for a more general discussion of helping young children with a variety of communication difficulties, which is beyond the scope of this chapter.) The therapist needed to view communication with Patrick as a total activity, deliberately seeking ways both verbally and non-verbally to encompass and address Patrick's severe limitations in language and in experiences with adults in close relationships. She also needed to help him to clarify and understand his current feelings and thoughts, which had been distorted and damaged by abuse.

Part of the therapist's skill in communication lies in accurately and acutely perceiving sometimes even small gestures and changes in orientation by a child which are indicative of his choices and wishes; an example is Patrick's shift of gaze in his early sessions to a toy he wanted but was too anxious to get in more direct ways. Behavioural cues, which include smaller gestures, eye movement and, of course larger actions, feature large in young children's communications. The therapist must not only be highly alert to and focused on the child's total communication, she must also translate her own communications into messages that the young child can readily understand. By making deliberate and extensive use of 'emotive messages', which Heard and Lake (1986) define as communications which are both verbal and non-verbal, and include tones of voice, gestures and facial expressions, the therapist becomes more able to convey her own feelings and thoughts concerning the child's responses and behaviour. Unlike therapeutic communications with older children and adults, the therapist must repeatedly and deliberately link her emotive messages to her highly visible, larger motor actions. The child can understand these actions more easily and can immediately see them as being directly responsive to his signals. Patrick's distaste over feeling sand on his hands, for instance, was responded to by the therapist, and his feelings acknowledged by her voice tone and facial expression of disgust while she looked steadily at his hands. This was immediately followed by her clearly altered voice tone of relaxed pleasure, concentration on her own hands and a purposeful, overt gesture, very obvious to Patrick, in which she brushed sand from her own hands. She accompanied these communications with the appropriate verbal message that sand was not a substance which she found disturbing.

From this example it can be seen that, given Patrick's limited language ability, the therapist could not have communicated this complex message to Patrick simply through talking to him. Her communications with Patrick were in some ways similar to those she used with Anna in chapter 4, who was largely silent in her sessions. The therapist had to pay attention to small details of both Anna's and Patrick's behaviour, and keep her communications on a non-threatening level in order to decrease their anxiety within therapy sessions. Both children were highly sensitive to small non-verbal reactions in the therapist and very alert to the therapist's reactions to them in turn. However, Anna, unlike Patrick, was selectively mute in her play sessions; she was intelligent, more experienced and more mature, and was therefore able to understand far more complex verbal messages from the therapist. Patrick's language ability was reported at referral to be at a rudimentary level for a four-year-old child, which was confirmed for the therapist in her therapeutic work with him. Language did nonetheless have an important role to play in Patrick's session too.

Language skills in working with young children

In general, as we have discussed in our earlier book (Wilson et al., 1992), a therapist adapts her language usage to the level the child speaks and understands. Guided by her experience of normal language usage, the therapist's language slightly advances and normalises the child's own usage, as examples from Patrick's sessions illustrate. As an American working in an English setting, the therapist may also need to adapt her speech for the children she works with, in order both to be understood and to reduce children's anxiety concerning her 'strangeness'. Given ethnic and regional linguistic variations, all therapists will to some extent need to make these deliberate strategic adjustments to their normal speech in working with different children. With younger children and developmentally delayed children like Patrick, this adjustment by the therapist is more acute because of the children's restricted understanding of language, a restriction which arises both because of their developmental stage and because their language is more likely to be limited to language levels used within their families.

In order to increase her language skills, it is useful for the therapist to listen carefully to the way in which the carer talks to the child, as the therapist consciously did with Patrick and Louise. Studying video and audio recordings of early sessions in detail and playing back unclear passages is also helpful in tuning in to a child's usual speech patterns, the therapist's replies and areas of miscommunication. If a child's speech is particularly unclear as a result of impairment or developmental delay, the therapist will be reliant on the carer as a source of information on the child's vocabulary and, when necessary, as a direct translator. We do not think, on the other hand, that the therapist should be too conscientious in attempting to decipher each word the child produces. As long as the child and therapist understand each other's main verbal messages, and the child does not become too frustrated in the process of communicating thoughts and feelings, it is more useful to concentrate on choosing simple words and structures, together with non-verbal ways of conveying meaning to the child. (An overabundance of questions about language, as with other kinds of questions, can in fact unintentionally convey the opposite message, that the therapist is not responsive to the child.) There are already many different levels of skills to focus on, and even experienced therapists can risk mental overload. Finally, the therapist need not understand each word the young child produces nor the child completely understand the therapist's utterances. This is because with young children an important part of their language development involves adapting their idiosyncratic speech to others and widening their range of language comprehension to include people outside their family.

The therapist's role differs from the speech therapist's, since the main purpose of therapy is not to advance the child's acquisition of language. Yet, as we have seen with Patrick, the enlargement of a young child's language capacity often occurs as an indirect result of non-directive play therapy because the environment of the playroom provides what is thought by psycholinguists to be an ideal environment for early language acquisition. That is, first of all, words are linked directly by the adult to the child's own emotions and actions; second, the adult's responses are at a slightly more advanced level than the child is generally capable of producing; and third, the environment is free from extraneous interruptions and distractions from the adult/child interactions.

One of the primary skills of the play therapist, as we have said often, is to reflect a child's ongoing feelings accurately. One way in which the child's language and thinking will hopefully be enriched is in the area of emotional expressions and emotional understanding. To help her reflections of feelings, the therapist needs to have a knowledge of how to translate more complex emotions and experiences of a young child into simple phrases within his or her potential vocabulary. The therapist also requires knowledge of children's normal and abnormal emotional development. As well as awareness of general trends in children's normal emotional development (see Wilson et al., 1992, chapter 5, for one general theoretical structure for understanding emotional development, that of Erikson), the therapist's practice can be helped by recent psychological interest and research in children's theory of mind. Investigations include research on children's emotional understanding of social and personal events (see, for example, Dunn, 1988; Harris, 1989; Wellman, 1990). We have also developed a general underlying framework for therapists to clarify their own thinking about the relation of emotion to thought and action in children in our earlier book.

With a child such as Patrick, the therapist's expectations of his capacity to experience basic emotional reactions, including surprise, interest, happiness, fear, anger and sadness (Lewis et al., 1989) will help her develop appropriate emotive messages, with a vocabulary within Patrick's understanding. Deep happiness, for instance, was reflected to Patrick verbally by: 'You're *so pleased* Louise's here again, Patrick!' (The therapist made use of British understatement of strong emotion here, recognising Patrick's probable familiarity with this specific linguistic usage of 'so pleased', simultaneously conveying very strong emotion to him with her voice tone and facial expression, and arms slightly stretched outward towards himself and Louise. With an American child, on the other hand, the therapist would probably have said 'very excited' or 'very happy' instead.) Another example is Patrick himself using the word 'bad' to convey both fear and anger in his statement: 'Big toilet bad!' This term was then extended together with more verbal emphasis by the therapist: 'You think it's *very bad* for you ...'

In non-directive play therapy, then, the therapist attempts to reflect the child's thoughts and feelings at the child's level of understanding. With young children the therapist will be using reflective skills which are somewhat different from those used with older children and adults, especially educated adults. Therapists working at this more advanced linguistic level (see for example, Siegelman, 1990) often find that literature and poetry are essential aids for the study of and enrichment of their own emotional repertoire and language. For children with very limited language development, however, the problem is somewhat different, as we have seen. The therapist needs to ask what emotional capacities and what vocabulary the young child will have to work with, and learn to scale down the richness of adult vocabulary to basic words and phrases, combined in ways that are unique for each child's life experiences. In addition, the totality of the communications between therapist and child needs to be thought about, and the therapist's language must be supplemented with many more explicit, action-based non-verbal emotive messages.

Responding to allegations of abuse made during therapy

Another related practice issue for the therapist with a child who has only rudimentary verbal communication is that the therapist must guard against overinterpretation of both the verbal and especially the non-verbal content of the child's communications. Take, for instance, Patrick's verbal statement to the therapist while he was clutching his genitals that his mother and father hurt him. The therapist could justifiably hypothesise that Patrick's action signified a behavioural memory of his sexual abuse, both because of the likelihood that children retain behavioural memories of abuse (see chapter 7) and because of his earlier allegations. But sometimes young children, and male children in particular (Newson and Newson, 1968; Grocke, 1991), hold their genitals when excited. Therefore the therapist had also to consider this as a possible, although less likely explanation. The therapist, aware of these alternatives, tried to convey to Patrick a factual account of his behaviour, rather than suggesting a causal sequence to him. She therefore joined his action and words together with the statement: 'They hurt you a lot. You're holding yourself there' (looking at his genital area). Patrick himself then explicitly linked his hurt with his penis.

The therapist herself had refrained from labelling his genital area as 'wee-wee', although she had made certain to check on Patrick's and his carers' terminology for his genitals and other body parts at her referral meetings. There were several reasons for her caution. Patrick might, as we have said, have been clutching his genitals because he was excited, in which case linking this act to the statement about his parents hurting him would have been confusing to him. In addition, young children are not at times able to differentiate the exact bodily location of an injury in which the pain diffuses to other parts of the body. Another factor which resulted in caution was the therapist's knowledge that children who have been repeatedly abused may have multiple memories they are trying to convey in one action. With children who may have been sexually abused, the details surrounding their abuse may only gradually become known (Glaser and Frosh, 1988). Too specific labelling of actions or areas of the child's body by the therapist at an initial allegation may inhibit the further unfolding of this process for the child. It is very important therapeutically, as we have seen with the children in this book, that the child is the one to bring the unique memories to the surface of consciousness and, with the help of the therapist, deal with them.

A young child's behavioural cues, then, although potentially subject to misinterpretation, can also be used advantageously, as in Patrick's case, to help the therapist by drawing her attention to the bodily sources of the child's memories. This enables her to make links for the child in his or her integration of sensations, actions, thoughts and emotions connected with earlier and recent abusive experiences. We shall discuss this issue further in Ben's story (chapter 7).

In recent years there has been an emphasis in child protection work on careful, non-leading questions by the adult when interviewing children about their possible abuse (Jones, 1990; Home Office, 1992). This emphasis has concurrently been criticised as being dominated by legal and evidential considerations, and a concern with adult rights, paying insufficient attention to the needs of child victims. These criticisms seem to have some justification. In addition, investigative interviewing of children can be applied by professionals as an automatic, procedural requirement in abuse investigations, rather than being based on the child's capacities and emotional needs. Nevertheless, this concern with witness suggestibility has been fruitful in drawing all child care professionals' attention to the need for careful, non-leading questioning of children in allegations of abuse. It is also now better recognised by therapists and other professionals that therapeutic suggestions – or any other influential suggestions from other sources impinging on a person emotionally – can jeopardise either a child's or an adult's true memory for a personal event (Spencer and Flin, 1990). A 'false' or distorted memory for an emotionally important event may develop in such situations; or the person may harbour a sense of vagueness and self-doubt concerning his or her true memory for these events (Newson, 1990).

As we have discussed more fully elsewhere (chapter 7; Ryan and Wilson, 1995b), non-directive play therapy provides a viable therapeutic method which is both helpful to a child and largely free from suggestion. As we see with Patrick (and later with Delroy in chapter 5), the therapist does attempt to reflect the child's feelings and thoughts accurately, making verbal and more precise the images, thoughts and emotions which the child does not necessarily link together consciously himself. In that sense, non-directive therapy, similarly to other therapeutic techniques, is not 'suggestion-free' (as we discuss further in the chapter on Ben). But in non-directive play therapy, in contrast to other psychodynamic and more direct methods, the emphasis for the therapist is on current issues arising from the children themselves, on accurate reflection of their concerns and on minimal direct interpretation of their actions, feelings and thoughts. These features of a non-directive approach ensure that the accuracy of a child's genuine memory for past and more recent events is preserved within the therapeutic encounter. And, most importantly, this preservation of a child's memory for abusive events is based first of all on the *child's* therapeutic needs, but its secondary result is to serve the legal requirement of preserving the child's evidence from undue contamination and suggestion.

As we have seen here, the therapist's role when an allegation of abuse is made by a child during play sessions is to follow general child protection rules and report any abuse allegations to the social services department. In this case the therapist reported the child's statements to the child's social worker. (We have emphasised throughout that if the child appears to be in immediate danger, then the therapist needs to question the child more closely immediately to determine risk, and *must* therefore depart from the customary reflective therapeutic approach.) This agency will then decide which level and method of investigating the allegation is appropriate in a particular case. The therapist's opinion, as one of the prime professionals and in some cases the only professional, who has first-hand, relevant information on the child's psychological well-being and needs, should be solicited by the agency from the beginning of their investigation onwards.

Sometimes the therapist's opinion may be overlooked and the therapist then needs to make certain of being involved in the decision-making process from the outset (see Furness, 1991, on issues for interprofessional collaboration in abuse cases). At other times, the child protection agency may wish to overinvolve the therapist and co-opt her relationship with the child. An attempt may be made by the police, social workers or legal representatives to turn the therapist's next play sessions with the child into sessions which approximate, either to a small or to a large degree, an investigative interview situation. We do not feel we can make an absolute rule that further questioning of the child should not take place within the therapy sessions, because in some cases the collection of evidence is imperative if this child or another child is at grave risk of further abuse, or the community itself is in immediate danger. We do, however, believe that the therapeutic relationship should be used in this manner with the utmost caution. All the professionals involved in the case need first to think creatively of alternative investigative methods available to them, rather than, as sometimes occurs, viewing the child's therapy sessions as the least problematic and most accessible vehicle for the collection of evidence where there have been allegations of abuse. (See Jones and Krugman, 1986, for a discussion of the therapeutic difficulties involved in this kind of change of purpose).

In Patrick's case, given his age and his limited understanding of adult concerns with abuse, the therapist did not discuss at any length the possible ensuing investigative process with him. She simply mentioned to him her need to inform his social worker of what he said and waited for any verbal or non-verbal signs from Patrick immediately after her statement or later on which would indicate that this had been insufficient. Since Patrick seemed to accept what she had said easily, simply nodding and carrying on in a relaxed manner with his ongoing activity of pretending to bathe the doll, the therapist did not develop this issue further, as she might have done with an older child or with a child who had not readily accepted what she had said.

It may interest the reader to know that Patrick's social worker, Cathy, and her team manager, in collaboration with their legal representatives and the police, decided not to conduct a formal investigative interview with Patrick because his age, development and his emotional vulnerability would prevent him from being allowed to testify in a criminal court setting. For civil proceedings purposes, Cathy made an audiorecording of her conversation with him the next day on this topic at his foster home, in the presence of a colleague known to Patrick who took detailed notes. This evidence was later used in civil proceedings, where the judge made a ruling of fact concerning Patrick's sexual abuse by his parents.

In Patrick's sessions we again see several instances where the therapist was unable to understand the referents for his behaviour and remarks. He was very interested and concerned by what he viewed as a girl on the game box crying. Even though he was corrected gently by the therapist because she knew that young children generally need adult help in identifying pictorial expressions of emotion, Patrick still persisted in seeing the emotion as distress rather than surprise. The therapist in correcting his perception followed her general rule of trying to give a child accurate information, in this case about the portrayal of an emotion, but to do this in a way that did not negate Patrick's own experiences and perceptions. Patrick's lack of change in his perception after the therapist's remark did not appear to be due to a stubborn insistence on his own viewpoint or an inability to understand what the therapist was saying. Nor did it seem that he was simply inexperienced in deciphering emotional representations on pictures. Patrick's emotions, in the therapist's opinion, seemed to be skewing his perceptions. Patrick also seemed strongly affected, as seen in one of his later sessions, by having in the past seen a lady crying.

While his specific experience(s) were unknown to the therapist, she observed that Patrick seemed to take a strong interest in and to be affected by female reactions. The therapist recalled that she had been told that Patrick's parents had had a physically violent relationship, with the mother sometimes suffering from bruising and other facial injuries. She speculated (to herself, of course) that Patrick might have witnessed physical assaults on his mother by his father, or the after-effects of these assaults emotionally on the mother, and that this would account for his stronger interest in crying rather than more positive emotions in females and in children. It would also partially account for the inhibition of his own play and movements without adult permission. He could have been living with not only a fear of pain from his sexual abuse, but from a more general fear of physical violence against himself and his mother. Later on, when the therapist learned of Louise's impending hospitalisation, she also wondered if Patrick could have been influenced by the emotional climate in his foster home as well, feeling more anxiety about women suffering harm both because of Louise's apprehensions and his own worry about her.

Similarly, the therapist did not have precise information to explain Patrick's unusual emotional reaction of anxiety when she removed her shoes at his request during their play therapy session. She noted and reflected his fearfulness and gave him reassurances, again speculating to herself that his reaction might tie in to a specific memory of his in which an adult removed their shoes as a prelude to perhaps an abusive experience, becoming for Patrick a generalised anxious reaction: when an adult takes off their shoes and reveals their bare feet, something bad will happen. This emotional reaction of Patrick's could link in with other instances in his sessions which indicated that Patrick's early experiences were very disabling for him in his current life, inhibiting his normal functioning. In all the unclear instances which appeared emotionally important to Patrick, the therapist in general terms described his 'possible worries' about adults removing their clothing to Cathy and Louise in her progress meeting, without breaching the confidentiality of his sessions. However, they could not help her in clarifying the possible meanings of these play sequences; the specific referents for these sequences, therefore, remained unsolved, which inevitably lessened her certainty in responding appropriately to them.

Using other therapeutic skills and the therapeutic value of routines

Patrick's specific anxieties and the methods the therapist used in helping him to overcome them are examples of how the play therapist can use different therapeutic skills, in this case desensitisation techniques, within an overall non-directive context. By her awareness, for example, of 'fading', 'modelling' and 'mirroring', the non-directive therapist is able to employ these techniques at the child's pace and within the context of understanding and helping him with more complex emotional problems. She is also able to link a specific fear to other more pervasive fears and to a child's developmental delays, rather than employing desensitisation in its traditional manner as a more isolated, adult-led technique. (See Singer, 1994, for an example of toilet phobia.) The therapist is also able to coordinate her own work with the child within her sessions with approaches to the child from his school and home environment at timely, receptive moments in the child's therapeutic progress, rather than at the time when the adults alone may identify the child's fears as problematic.

Another feature of practical interest is the manner in which the therapist helped Patrick to create his own routines for his sessions. In our earlier book we have outlined and illustrated the therapist's detailed structuring of the sessions, for example, the needed consistency for the child around time, place, and the therapist's predictable responses and attitudes. We have also mentioned that the children themselves will attempt to establish their own routines within the sessions. Within a child's normal development, as we highlight in the next section on theoretical issues, young children automatically create routines for themselves and this propensity for routines feeds into the child's development of 'scripts' for everyday events which in time become incorporated into symbolic play. This routinisation of life events by a child occurs sometimes to the surprise of carers and is often developed by a child around new skills or around other somewhat stressful events. These routines, such as handing a young child the cup of his drink in a particular way, can be ones that the adult herself is originally unaware of, until the child himself becomes insistent on the 'right' procedure. In play therapy, in order to make the session highly predictable and therefore emotionally safer because it is within the child's understanding and control, the therapist is able deliberately to keep to the same routine in beginning a session with the child (with minor variations). But as Patrick showed, young children also can be easily helped to evolve their own rituals which can then be respected by the therapist. With Patrick his routine beginning helped him to feel secure initially in the playroom, to feel a sense of ready familiarity when he came each time, and to feel less anxious when Louise was hospitalised and Steve brought him instead. For older children the routines are usually less detailed and less inflexible, consisting more of general procedures which help reduce their anxiety. But a few older children, such as Delroy in chapter 5, may need more adult guidance when their emotional and physical difficulties result in a lack of regularity and inhibition of their actions. In these cases the therapist herself will try to help them set up a routine, predictable beginning and ending for their sessions, as she would with a much younger child.

THEORETICAL ISSUE

Restoring a child's normal developmental trajectory within play therapy

In discussing practice issues connected with Patrick's play therapy in our previous section, we referred to ways in which the therapist needed knowledge of normal developmental processes in order to understand his responses and help him to correct and enhance his earlier distorted experiences. More broadly, it seems useful to view the therapist's purpose in non-directive play therapy as creating an artificial, more enhanced environment where children who have experienced damaging adult–child social interactions are able, through their interactions with the therapist, to re-experience and rework these experiences into more normal socialisation patterns (Ryan and Wilson, 1995a).

They are enabled to do this because, in non-directive play therapy, conditions are created which are similar to the optimum socialisation processes which occur between an infant and carer during normal development. These processes are intensified through the heightened conditions offered in therapy. In this section, we consider some of these and show, by discussing Patrick's therapy, the ways in which children can be helped to catch up on crucial early experiences which they have missed, or to change behaviours (such as fearfulness or timidity) which have resulted from damaging experiences. The conditions created in therapy are based on, and/or mimic, the kinds of experiences which infants would have with their carers in their earliest social interactions. Features of these kinds of normal social experiences within sessions include: the development of familiar, consistent routines based on a child's attachment needs; the encouragement of normal, age-appropriate exploratory behaviour through alertness to the child's cues and repetitive action on the therapist's part; the enhancement of the child's language learning environment (already referred to in the previous section); and the encouragement of the child's capacity for symbolic play, through playful exchanges and routines.

We have said above that the therapist needs to help a child to feel as secure as possible in a strange environment. Following attachment theory, which argues the need for a secure base from which the child can begin to explore the world (see chapter 6 for a fuller discussion), with security the child will then be more able to explore the room and equipment, and eventually the internal environment of feelings and thoughts, more readily. As well as trying to ensure that the adult bringing the child to sessions is regarded by him/her as reliable and stable – and hopefully emotionally receptive and available (see chapter 6 for mistakes in this respect) – the therapist also attempts to be highly dependable and predictable herself in her movements and to make the room itself predictably ordered, private and free from unexpected interruptions. The child is encouraged to become part of this predictability, being allowed by the therapist, as we saw with Patrick, to develop his own active routines within his sessions. This artificial enhancement of predictable features allows even very young and very anxious children to develop a sense of security more quickly and easily. It deliberately mimics some of the predictable features of the normal home play environment of a young child, while consciously enhancing and making more child-centred other aspects of the playroom.

This emphasis on a stable environment also has the effect of creating a static background which serves to heighten the child's and the therapist's ability to notice and respond to the child's internal thoughts and feelings, the child's external actions within the playroom and social interactions with the therapist. The therapist above all tries to be emotionally predictable to the child. This heightening of emotional predictability by the therapist seems particularly important for children whose emotional development has been significantly damaged or delayed. Ainsworth (1973) has described the activities of mothers of securely attached infants as being highly responsive to their infants; Murray (1989) and Stern (1985) also demonstrate the attunement and responsiveness necessary between a caregiver and infant for meaningful social interactions. The therapist, then, is mimicking the actions and attitudes of a sensitive caregiver to her child's needs.

In addition to being highly responsive and available emotionally to the child in their play sessions, the therapist uses the method of non-directive play therapy systematically and predictably to give an underlying therapeutic consistency to her attitudes and behaviour with the child. As Patrick demonstrates, an important component of this approach is for the therapist to allow the child to make genuine choices and to become aware of his own individual feelings in interactions with the therapist. This in turn helps him to develop greater competence in his own self-chosen activities and in social interactions with significant adults. Skills which are normally developed in infancy by repeated adult–infant communications can be developed or reworked by troubled, abused or emotionally neglected children through more intensive interactions with the therapist. Child–therapist interactions can help a child develop more appropriate face-to-face communications. For example, overly fearful children unable to meet the gaze of trustworthy adults may develop an ability to tolerate direct eye contact at appropriate times during social interactions during play sessions (Ryan and Wilson, 1995a). Also, at the other extreme, a child who demands constant adult attention and eye contact may develop the ability to engage in more autonomous activities out of sight of the therapist, learning to trust that significant adults 'think about' or carry internal images of the child's well-being and needs, even when that child is out of sight. This in turn helps the child reciprocally to develop benign and trusting internal models of adult care.

The therapist may also help a child develop less complex or distorted patterns of interactions into more normal ones. Patrick's early responses to the therapist were similar to those of a very young child who is unable to act himself on his environment and needs to have the caregiver respond to and act on his interest in objects in the immediate surroundings. Patrick remained rooted to the spot near the sandbox to which he had gone when he entered the room for his first session, and was unable spontaneously to move to another play object when his interest changed. The therapist needed to follow his eye movements, as a caregiver would do with an infant, to find out what was of interest to the infant before gestures and speech helped the infant communicate his wishes more clearly to others. Then the therapist rather than Patrick needed to take the initiative and get the game down from the shelf for him, even though it was within his reach. She also needed to check his non-verbal cues (nodding, gazing) to be certain she was correct, verbalising her actions and thoughts in basic language. There were many other times in their sessions when Patrick seemed to need the therapist to perform an action repeatedly for him while he watched intently, before venturing to perform that action himself. When the therapist pulled the sandy toys out of the sand, or brushed the sand off the toys for Patrick's use, or brushed the sand off her own hands, for instance, it seems possible that Patrick was having the therapist perform those actions in order to observe her closely. He later seemed to feel able to incorporate these normal actions into his own repertoire in more normal, age-appropriate play and social activities.

For the above reasons, the child's play sessions also seem to provide a child with an ideal language learning environment, again paralleling in a more intensive manner a caregiver's input with a child. Schaffer (1989) states, for example, that language development proceeds more quickly for a young child when the adult's language is 'related to the child's interests, attentional focus and actions at that moment. The mother therefore needs to be attuned to the child and tie her own comments with the child's concerns as well as with its abilities to process what she says' (quoted in Ryan and Wilson, 1995a). This is reflected in the therapist's function of using verbalisation or 'naming' experience to help a child understand what they are experiencing internally and externally.

Another feature of early development is the emergence of symbolic play. The infant uses playful social exchanges and routine, familiar give-and-take games between infant and carer as the basis for the beginnings of his or her rudimentary symbolic play (Ryan and Wilson, 1995a). In normal development, the carer often takes the lead and adapts an infant's routine, more basic play activity, say chewing on a dummy, into another kind of playful, reciprocal activity between them, for example, the carer playfully putting the dummy into her own mouth *pretending* that she herself is the child, and then encouraging the child to offer it to her. This type of reciprocal exchange is similar to the actions of the therapist and Patrick with the baby bottle, except that Patrick, being capable of more actions and initiative himself than an infant would be, took the lead himself in imitating a carer's behaviour, but in a largely unconscious way. Like a young child's carer, the therapist sensed that Patrick too needed support and encouragement from her to develop this social exchange into a new and more advanced level of symbolic play.

Patrick's great hesitation and uncertainty in taking up this kind of play, together with his usual concrete level of play and his rapid advancement in symbolic play during his later sessions, all imply that his earlier experiences had in all probability hindered him from developing this type of play at its normal time and in its usual manner. When children have an over-ripeness for an essential stage in their development because of an emotionally impoverished or neglectful environment or physical constraints, they often make unusually rapid advances in a subsequent, enriched environment. Many examples are called to mind – Helen Keller's use of signing, the slum children in Montessori's early work, or, more recently, infants and children from Romanian orphanages who were understimulated and significantly developmentally delayed, and yet have made very rapid progress following their adoption. Patrick's rapid progression in symbolic play began with an initial role play of himself as the carer and the therapist as the child which was very one-sided, with the therapist performing most of the actions. However, Patrick quickly enlarged his understanding of symbolic play and applied it soon to many different situations himself. His foster carers also reported that he had a new eagerness for more advanced play with them at home.

In looking closely at these leaps in development which occur for children who have been developmentally delayed, clues and hypotheses about the essential features of the environment and of the child which must be present in order to unlock this stage of development for children can be teased out. Fraiberg's (1977) research on blind children's delays in physical milestones such as crawling and walking has informed us of the importance of object targets for such activities in normal development and demonstrated the ways in which more abstract thought is necessary for auditory and tactile compared to visual targets. In the same way work with children such as Patrick in non-directive play therapy can give pointers and help us develop research hypotheses on essentials for the development of symbolic play. In addition to the child requiring one-to-one social interactions with a person (in most cultures normally an adult or an older child), the person also seems to need to attend to the child's responses and modulate his or her own activities in accordance with the child's interests. Children also seem to have to perceive the situation as one in which their physical needs have been met (and with older children who have a history of poor parenting, to feel that future needs will also be adequately met), allowing them to relax their attention from their immediate needs. The child will also have to be capable of at least the limited level of cognitive functioning in which it is possible to place oneself in another's role, which happens in normal development by about 18 months of age.

There also seem to be certain characteristics of symbolic play itself which a child needs to learn in social interactions. One feature of normal play described in the play research literature and which was evident in Patrick's sessions was that children seem to have distinctive ways of marking out for their play audience and partners that their behaviour is a play production (Bretherton, 1984). Several verbal and non-verbal 'metacommunications', which serve the purpose for play sequences of conveying to others how to respond to and interpret words and actions, have been identified by Giffin (1984). One very basic, immediately understood non-verbal communication used by the therapist with Patrick was frequent smiling and laughter — the therapist was conveying that what they were doing was *fun*. Patrick had already spontaneously erupted in giggles during his more concrete pouring activities with juice and the therapist was showing him that their next shared activity was now fun for her and indicating that it could be pleasurable for both of them. The therapist was also showing Patrick that the usual activity at the beginning of a play sequence is to clarify the players' roles (e.g. 'Maybe I'm a baby'). Imitating her behaviour would lead Patrick to develop this normal play device of establishing roles at the outset of a play sequence for himself in later symbolic play sequences inside and outside the playroom. (The therapist, of course, was also demonstrating to Patrick that she was able to be directed by him and responsive to his signals.)

The therapist was using the play devices of stereotypic depiction of roles and overacting (e.g. 'Waah! Where's my bottle?', then making sucking noises followed by satisfied ones while drinking), as well as changing her voice register to another key. The therapist in using these devices was attempting to show Patrick that he could play out with her a play 'script' of a carer attending to the baby's needs. As play research has demonstrated, normal play of young children can be classified in terms of 'scripts' which are based on real-life shared events (Bretherton, 1984). These scripts have early beginnings in carer–child interactions (Newson and Newson, 1979; Bruner, 1983) and later evolve into scripts which are shared in common with play partners by preschool children based on similar personal experiences, such as 'it's going to be my birthday party and you come' and shared fantasies, such as 'pretend you're the bride . . .'. Early scripts, such as Patrick's first attempt with the bottle, commonly seem to be both brief and based on real events in a child's life.

Another feature of normal play, in which the players, while enacting and experiencing the already established script, then further develop and explore their ensuing actions together, is labelled by Giffin (1984) as 'ulterior conversation', as we see in the next chapter with Diane. Other within-play communications, such as the therapist's remarks to Patrick about 'just playing' and it being 'very odd' to see her drinking, serve to ground the child's play experience in reality. Although these seem to be very rudimentary and largely the job of the adult in early symbolic play, they nonetheless still appear to be an important feature of early symbolic play enactments.

Once play scripts are established, the child in play therapy whose play has been developmentally delayed will often quickly begin to use these scripts more flexibly and in a much less rudimentary manner. For example, in his next sessions Patrick extended his symbolic play to using the figures in the doll's house. (The therapist checked with Louise, when talking to her about ways in which to extend the range of Patrick's play, that he had not to her knowledge ever exhibited these more advanced levels of play at home.) Again his play was initially simple, using the figures to represent foster family members and himself in routine activities at home. But once Patrick was able to play on this symbolic level, the therapist in turn was able to have greater scope and flexibility in helping him to express his troubled emotions and earlier experiences, the most noteworthy example being his reference to the toilet and his sexual abuse by his parents. She was also able to help him express his current feelings and think about his ongoing experiences more fully, which seemed as he played out these scripts to increase his feelings of security and sense of belonging in his foster family.

Finally, Patrick's play demonstrates how rapidly, once he was engaged in non-directive play therapy and once his new level of symbolic enactment of life experiences was activated, he was able to move on to use this means in order to work through his troubling current experiences. He had a more flexible and deeper way to express his insecurity and anxiety when Louise was hospitalised than he would have had at the beginning of his therapy. At first in this particular session Patrick acted out his distress physically by attempting to hit the playroom window. However, once the therapist recognised his feelings, set safe limits to his behaviour and calmed him with her receptive manner, Patrick relaxed and tried out some rudimentary symbolic play in which he symbolised the play cushion as a bag (in retrospect a prelude to his using the 'bag' in a more extensive symbolic capacity) and performed the reciprocal physical action with the therapist of rolling the cushion back and forth playfully, as they had done earlier with the ball.

Patrick was then able, after this 'warm-up', to enact a much more advanced symbolic play sequence than he had previously exhibited. Patrick's cognitive capacities seemed to rise suddenly to this all-important task and he developed the play situation himself into one in which the therapist was the child (again – and the most usual early role reversal) and he himself was Louise leaving with her bag and then returning to the child. Patrick needed to repeat this play sequence twice more, until, it seemed, he had been reassured by the identical ending each time that Louise would return home to him. (She had told him verbally about this repeatedly, and even left him her handbag, as the therapist had suggested, in order to allay Patrick's strong fear of abandonment, which, given his attachment history, was to be anticipated.) It should not be overlooked, however, that despite a young child's new-found ability to play out anxiety symbolically, this mental coping strategy is usually still used sparingly by the child and needs always to be in conjunction with direct, physical reassurance from the carer. The therapist recognised Patrick's need, and helped him to build upon the sense of coping and hopefulness which had developed in him during their play session, by allowing him to return easily to Steve's care when he was ready to end the session.

The rapid development of Patrick's capacity to engage in symbolic play during his play therapy sessions came to include his ability to use his play symbolically to end his time with the therapist by placing her at the far end of the room and playing alone. We hope this chapter has shown the way in which children can both redress their emotionally difficult and abnormal life experiences and also develop more normal symbolic play patterns in play therapy, which can then rapidly be expanded and applied to coping with current life events. Older children, as we see next with Diane, have usually developed a much more advanced level of symbolic play. However, the basic interaction patterns between adult and child seen in Patrick's emerging symbolic play may still be lacking or distorted. The therapist will then work at the older child's more advanced level of play, with metacommunications and other features of symbolic play being used as vehicles to help a child (re)establish normal developmental trajectories.

Chapter 3

Diane
Repairing and Creating Identity

> *might I, if you can find it, be given*
> *a chameleon with tail*
> *that curls like a watch spring; and vertical*
> *on the body – including the face – pale*
> *tiger stripes, about seven;*
>
> Marianne Moare 'Saint Nicholas'

Diane was ten years old when I first met her; a child of medium height and rather heavy build, with auburn hair, pale freckled cheeks and a way of holding her head down so that her hair fell forward over her eyes. She had been in care for nearly a year when her social worker contacted me and asked if I could help with the problems that she still seemed to be experiencing both at school and in her foster home. From talking to her foster mother, class teacher and social worker, I learned something of her early experiences, and why it was felt that she needed further help.

Diane and her younger brother, Jason, now aged eight, were brought up by their mother and father until their father left home when Diane was seven. Although not a lot is known about these early years, Diane's parents seem to have had a stormy relationship, and Diane's mother, Carole, as the social worker put it, was 'very much up and down – one minute all over the children and the next minute yelling at them for no obvious reason', so one may guess that life for the children was even then pretty turbulent.

Soon after Diane's father had departed, Carole seems to have become very depressed and herself left home, leaving the children alone in the house, where they were discovered by neighbours and then taken into care. She returned after a week and the children went back to live with her, but she left home three or four times again over the next 18 months, with the children going backwards and forwards between home and foster care. Finally, Diane's school noticed that her arms and legs were covered in bruises, and her mother admitted to having kicked and punched her. Carole was convicted of assault and the children were again received into care, and this time placed with their present foster carers, where they had been ever since.

Supervised contact was arranged in order to try and help mother, father (who had now returned home) and children get back together again. The children became overexcited during these visits, and the parents tended to over-react, becoming angry, shouting, and the father even cuffing Jason on one occasion when he cried. The children were distressed afterwards, apparently having been made to feel that they were to blame for being in care and that in order to go home they needed to be good (rather than their parents needing to try too). No final decision had been taken about their future, but it had been decided, with the court's agreement, to suspend the visits for a while because the children became so upset. A family therapist had tried to work with the parents, but Carole had declined further contact after the first couple of sessions, and the children's father had maintained that it was not his problem and refused from the outset to participate.

The adults involved in looking after Diane were worried about her because she seemed so passive and shut in on herself when with them. At school, she seemed listless and lacking in energy, and was either picked on or ignored by the other children. At home, she used to try to take charge of Jason, and seemed to enjoy playing with him when he was amenable to her instructions. However, if he showed independence, Diane had short outbursts of rage at him and then withdrew into herself.

It was agreed that I would work with Diane initially for six, hourly, sessions once a week for a short-term assessment of her therapeutic needs for the court. (See final chapter for a discussion of this kind of assessment, which is outside the scope of this chapter.) Further funds became available near the end of this assessment period and an additional nine sessions were conducted. Diane's use of play therapy also seemed to deepen significantly after this turning point in her sessions.

I first met Diane and her foster carers at home. I explained how we would be working and arranged that Diane would come to the playroom with her foster carer the following week.

DIANE'S PLAY THERAPY SESSIONS

Work in play therapy seldom proceeds in a tidy sequence, since different themes often emerge in play, disappear for a while and then reappear as the child reactivates them. However, looking back on Diane's sessions they did seem to divide into a beginning phase (the first to fifth sessions), a middle phase (from the sixth to the twelfth) and a final phase in the last three sessions.

We shall describe these three phases of Diane's play therapy and at the end of each of the phases briefly discuss the key themes which emerged. The section on practice issues which follows will first consider the ways in which role-playing may be used by the child in non-directive play therapy, along with practice concerns for the therapist in responding to and participating in such role-plays. The second practice issue is a consideration of ways to evaluate therapeutic progress. This will be discussed particularly in relation to Diane's play therapy, although evaluation is also touched on in many of the other chapters of the book (for example the chapters on Patricia and Anna). Finally, the theoretical section of this chapter will consider physical abuse, its impact on the child, and how the problems which arise from it are addressed in play therapy.

In the first phase of play therapy some of the problem areas in Diane's life were touched on, and she explored her feelings about being good and being naughty, showing her need for adult approval and her anxieties about adult censure if she was untidy. She touched fleetingly at this stage on her mixed feelings towards her younger brother, Jason, but this theme emerged more emphatically in the second phase, along with some of her even more intimate and difficult feelings, which centred on her relationship with her mother. In the final sessions, she continued to work on these themes, but also recapitulated earlier issues, as if preparing herself for the end of her play therapy.

First phase

At the beginning of her first session, Diane seemed subdued and did not look directly at me, moving instead immediately to the box of dressing up clothes and beginning to try on different costumes. However, she did not seem unduly anxious and, as she settled on a Red Indian costume and briefly admired herself in the mirror, she asked where all the clothes came from. Then, smiling at herself and trying out quiet 'whooping' noises, wondered, 'What do we come here for?' I replied: 'I was going to talk to you about that again. When we met last week I said that I work with children who have had a lot of things happening to them. They come to see me and they can talk and play with things, and I can help them work out some of the problems they have. Remember, I'll write about what you need to the judge.'

Diane did not respond to this, trying on another costume, so I commented that maybe she didn't want to listen to what I was talking about. 'I'm a policewoman with an Indian head-dress, a silly one', she responded and giggled. 'Now I'm a witch.' She hummed the tune from the Addams family. 'They're friendly', I commented. 'Yeah', she agreed.

Diane asked if she should put the things away and then if she could do some painting. I replied: 'I don't mind, it's for you to choose. You have an hour to do what you want. Some time to just do what you want and think about what you want.' As she painted, I continued: 'I try not to ask children what they want to talk about and what they want to do because I know a lot of people have been asking what you feel about things, about your mother and your father. I said I'd work with you and if you wanted to talk about that you could talk about it, but if you didn't that's all right as well. Have time for yourself.'

When she had finished painting, she made a point of putting the other clothes on the floor away but chose to dress up again in the Indian costume. She wanted to go and show her carer how she looked; I acknowledged that she was disappointed, that it would be nice to show her, but we stayed in here during the hour. Diane looked slightly crestfallen then began to use the limit creatively by making the video camera into an audience, and deciding to make a sequence on video of herself as a Red Indian. As she danced, whooping and beating a drum in front of the camera, I remarked, 'You feel like a real Indian.' 'I *am* a real Indian', she replied, seriously. I said: 'You're not a girl now; you're *real*, an Indian.'

Diane eagerly asked if she could watch her video. I readily agreed, but reminded her that we had only an hour and we'd have to watch it during that time. Diane watched the video with her face shining with pleasure. I briefly remarked, in order not to distract her, that she was excited by how she looked. Diane nodded vigorously, without taking her eyes off the monitor.

In the second session, she began by dressing up again, first as a witch, coating her face with dark green and black face paint, but then almost immediately rejecting this character and again making herself up as a Red Indian, developing a long dance and drum sequence. She watched it absorbedly again on the monitor and tried to negotiate a longer viewing time, which I had to refuse, with regret.

Diane's next two sessions were intensely messy ones. She began painting a face on a balloon, then completely covered the balloon with layers of paint, splattering the paint on with a brush and eventually with her hands. As she became more excited, she tossed the balloon in the air, asking me to bat it back and forth with her, rubbing her hands together and singing 'squishy-squashy' to herself as she threw the balloon back to me. I joined in, commenting that she wanted to have it all messy *and* to play with it, but I also insisted that we hit it gently enough to keep it at the uncarpeted end of the playroom. Diane then said 'I should give it a name', and called it 'Slob', started to tell it off when it was about to roll on to the carpet, tapping it and kicking it for its bad behaviour. After kicking it, she added anxiously and incongruously, 'He won't hurt you.' I agreed, saying that the balloon was just messy but that no-one would get hurt, and reassuring her that the room could be cleaned at the end of her session.

At the beginning of her fourth session, I reminded Diane that we had two times together after today, as we'd agreed. (I had requested, but not heard, whether further funding could be made available.) Diane quickly covered another balloon with paint and became very aggressive, banging the balloon repeatedly with the paint brush so that the paint splattered. I remarked that she seemed quite cross, right after I had said we didn't have much time left together. Diane silently recoated the balloon, smoothing it with her hands, and hit it again, repeating this sequence several times. I commented as she faintly smiled to herself that she wanted to have fun now. But I also began to check her actions when the paint started to splatter the walls. 'You're cross and excited, both together maybe, but you can't be *too* wild in here.' Winding down, Diane decided to play in the sand. When I reminded her that she needed to wash her hands first, she moved to the other end of the playroom, saying defiantly, 'I hate washing my hands.'

> V: Yes, it looks like you really don't want to. But you do want to play. You need to wash them first.
> V: [as she finally began to wash them] I think you like to be messy sometimes.
> D: [in a belligerent tone] Yes, *all* the time.
> V: You feel cross with me. In here you can be messy, but it's still not enough.'

Diane then started a game of stirring up all the sand in the sand tray with a spoon, which she played very energetically until she seemed exhausted. Yet she refused to stop, and continued to play from a kneeling position. I talked about how she felt she had to rush through everything today, that she didn't have enough time and couldn't stop, even when she felt exhausted. She then became very languid, lying on the floor and only reluctantly taking my offered hand and getting up when it was time to go. I found out later that Diane had been told off by her foster carer for throwing things around the waiting room before she'd come in to me.

She began her next, fifth, session in a subdued manner, playing in the sand box with her head well down and not looking at me. I said that she seemed very quiet; I had felt quiet earlier too, because I thought it was to be our next to last time today. But her social worker had called me yesterday to say that he had been given permission for us to have ten more sessions. I thought this was a very good idea, ten more after today. We could talk about what she thought and what I intended to say to the judge about what she needed now or another time, if she wanted to.

Diane listened and seemed deliberately to avoid replying by becoming more purposeful and busy in the sand. I added that I now knew she'd been in trouble for messing up the waiting room last time. I wished I'd told her our first time together that the rules we had in the playroom were different from most other places, including the waiting room. And even in the playroom, I did tell her where in the playroom she could be messy. Diane had become tense and alert in her stooped position over the sand. She was now visibly relaxed, complaining that her arm was hurting. 'You can think about your arm now and how you feel.' Getting a chair, she started including me in her sand play, making a large hideout on an island surrounded by the sea. The island sheltered Diane and her friends from their enemies. These enemies ended up fighting each other outside the hideout, leaving Diane and her friends in peace. At the end of this play sequence, she again settled on playing the musical instruments and watching them with me on the video monitor. As she left, she walked ahead, throwing the remark back to me that she had decided to come back *lots* of times.

Discussion of the first phase of Diane's play therapy

Diane's excitement and animation, which she showed in dressing up, suggested that there were many strong feelings that she felt unable to experience herself because of the need to be good and unobtrusive in order to please adults. It seems likely that Diane frequently felt colourless and unnoticed because she tried continually to be good and to please adults. The play therapist, in accepting these actions, was also giving Diane permission to be untidy, hoping to link untidiness with fun instead of always with naughtiness.

By wanting to show her carer the transformation in her appearance while playing, Diane also conveyed her need for more adult recognition of her strong feelings and of her personal importance. However, the imposition of the usual therapeutic limit of not leaving the room helped her focus on her actions inside the room in a more intensive way, and to confirm for herself her changed appearance and actions, rather than immediately turning to adults for acknowledgment and approval of them. By not praising Diane for any of her actions, the therapist also ensured that her search for adult approval was not continued excessively. Equally, the absence of any response suggesting either praise *or* blame helped to establish a therapeutic atmosphere of permissiveness, in which

Diane could be free to select those activities which she needed to in order to explore feelings which were salient for her.

In Diane's third session, she explored her feelings about messiness more intensively, and by having an inanimate object, the balloon, get into trouble and get hurt for being messy, she seemed to be trying out feelings that were threatening for her by placing them onto the balloon.

Just before Diane's fourth session, she had, as the therapist later discovered, been in trouble for making a mess in the waiting room, which she had then refused to clear up. This produced a short setback in her progress in therapy because, instead of reworking past feelings linking messiness with blame and punishment, she experienced this link directly in her current life. (Her behaviour was most probably linked strongly to her feeling of anger over her sessions finishing too soon.) Two mistakes seem to have been made: the therapist should have talked to Diane earlier about the permissiveness of the playroom and the difference between the way in which she could behave there compared to other settings. (The therapist mistakenly thought Diane was old enough to understand this difference herself and did not make a direct statement to her, as she would have done with a younger child.) Second, it is vital that adults who care for children attending therapy are sensitive to possible conflicting and confused behaviours or feelings which may become intensified in a child during therapy. The therapist, arguably, should have alerted Diane's foster carers to this conflict so that Diane's possible confusion could have been addressed by them more productively. This is not to say that Diane's misbehaviour in the waiting room should have gone unchecked, but the foster carer could have been encouraged to set a more appropriate limit, and to acknowledge Diane's feelings as she waited. By talking about what had happened the previous week, the therapist did seem accurately to reflect Diane's feeling of distress and to re-establish a sense of therapeutic safety, so that she was able to commit herself fully to the offer of further sessions.

Diane's middle sessions

Diane's next two sessions resembled each other somewhat in content. For her sixth session she entered the playroom carrying a toy trumpet, which she had brought from downstairs, and made a beeline for the dressing up clothes, announcing that she had to get ready. Posing in front of the camera, she announced that she was going to watch the video all through today. 'Now we're going to do some music', she said, standing in front of the video and blowing the trumpet, 'You think I'm good at it? I just made it up. Now we're going to try another one', and she showed me how she wanted me to sing while she played. 'Now I'm going to do face painting, then I'm going to do some dancing.' Diane placed the mirror so that she could look at herself, commenting that she had her hair up so that it wouldn't go in her face. She again decided to dress up as an Indian, but then applied heavy make-up – red lipstick, red and blue eyeshadow, and heavy pink blusher – to her face, rather than Indian warpaint. She deliberated over which hat to wear, rejecting several after trying them on and scrutinising her appearance in the mirror, finally choosing a small neat hat. She then devised another dance sequence in front of the camera, slowly marching round and ending with her feet stretched out on a cushion, smiling up at the camera. We watched it on the video, Diane commenting under her breath as we looked, 'It's good, that.'

At the beginning of the next (seventh) session, Diane complained that her head ached, and then immediately got the witch's hat from the box, saying to herself 'What else?', in a deep voice, and growling into the mirror. I said, 'You're starting to growl. I think you're one of those mean growling characters'. Diane began carefully to make up her face as a witch with black face paint, green eyes and lips. She wished 'everyone' could see her, as she started to blow the trumpet loudly, dance round the room, and ask for more instruments, getting me to clap in order to make more noise.

Diane then decided on a role-play and from this point onwards, role-playing became the principal vehicle which she used to work through her traumatic feelings and life experiences. Directing me in my role ('You say to me, go and wash your face you horrible girl'), she devised a complicated story, in which I became the mother who told her daughter that she would 'beat her in' for wearing make-up. The mother made Diane wash her face; she pretended to be frightened of her mother, but was secretly waiting to take charge. I said, as Diane growled in a deep unnatural voice, 'Who are you? I was waiting for my little girl.' Diane grabbed me forcefully and as I whimpered and acted frightened, shouted out, 'I am the black witch. No one can attack me! Everyone will love *me*, not her. I can command everyone.' Diane then put a spell on her mother, who managed somehow to kill the witch and escape.

The mother was told to awaken from 'the dream'. She found her daughter in the room with her and had to try to keep secret from her daughter the spell she had been under and her killing of the witch. But the daughter then revealed her power and real identity to her mother, saying,

> D: I sat down here and I wanted some food. You got me the food and put poison in it. I ate it and I died. Poisoning your own daughter! But I managed to survive the poison. You're a killer and a liar!

Receiving her lines from Diane, the mother replied that she hadn't wanted her little girl to find out her secrets. Then Diane would always think her mother was powerful and good and would always obey her. Diane confronted her mother with her wickedness: 'You tricked me. How could you trick me?!' The mother quietly said that she was ashamed and Diane matter-of-factly forgave her, even starting to enjoy being with her mother again.

Diane and her mother then companionably played musical instruments together, with Diane explaining that they were doing it because it might cheer her mother up. Reconciled, they play together, still in role as mother and daughter, Diane explained her actions: what happened was the only way she could 'get back at' the mother for being ordered to clean the mess off her face. I replied, 'So really it was the only way you could tell me that you were angry with me. You had to get back at me in such a bad way and we both hurt each other when we were angry. Then you found out everything.'

I dropped the toy recorder accidentally at this point, intent on my dialogue in role, and we both laughed. I said: 'We can still have fun together, can't we? Friends again?', and Diane nodded.

'Shall we play that story again?' Diane asked at the beginning of her next session, but digressed first deciding to make a Christmas card for her foster carer. Afterwards Diane altered the role-play by dressing up as a little boy and giving me the role of the older sister. The little boy was unreasonable, pushing the sister, then falling down and blaming her because he was hurt. The boy would run away, then want to play again while the sister remarked that he didn't know what he wanted. She tried to care for him, getting a drink and blanket, but the little boy sneaked out and got physically attacked and injured badly. The sister wanted to ask a grown up for help, but her brother refused and limped off to bed, where he lay very still. The sister was very worried and afraid, but the boy said not to call a doctor or any adults because they're all witches, 'even mum, she's probably a witch'. Once he was well again, the older sister tried desperately to keep her brother safe and happy by playing with him, keeping him quiet and giving him whatever he wanted. This was the only way she knew to help him. Diane ended the story at this point and, retrieving the Christmas card, took it with a very grave face to give to her foster mother.

During the following session (the ninth), Diane again devised a role-play involving herself and her younger brother, which took up the entire hour. This time, it gradually became clear that I was to take the role of the younger brother and Diane was herself, enticing her brother into being naughty. They then felt forced to run away from home to escape their father's anger. Diane disguised them both with make-up, teasing her little brother for being made up like a girl and looking ridiculous (which I indeed did!). When they were on the run, the brother became very scared at night, trying to make sure his older sister stayed right with him, and thinking about how angry their mum and dad would be with them if they ever went home.

In her next session, after complaining of feeling nauseous and looking rather uneasy at the beginning of the hour, Diane at once asked whether we could continue 'that runaway game'. She gathered the things together which we'd had last time, and quickly built a den for herself and her brother. She fixed it up as cosily as she could, including painting a few pictures for the walls. After decorating the den, Diane decided to put paint on my face. (I allowed her to put the paint on my hand and arm instead.)
Diane was mildly disappointed, but continued her story.

> D: [vindictively, as she coated my arm] You look *nasty.*
> V: [as younger brother, feeling powerless and wishing someone would help me] Maybe you'll get into trouble for it.

Diane remained silent, aggressively slapping paint.

> V: [tremulously] I don't like it.
> D: [viciously] Nobody cares about children like you! They can't get us, and besides, Mum and Dad are going to leave town.

As Diane painted my arm with another layer of colour, she began to spray paint everywhere and stopped only momentarily when I told her it was too much.

> D: [defiantly] I'll paint my *own* face and my *own* clothes then.
> V: [firmly] You can paint your hand and arm and your apron, but *not* your face. That could sting you. They're powder paints and not for near your eyes.
> D: [aggressively swinging her brush] Then I'll paint the whole room.

There was already more than enough paint to clean up in the last ten minutes of the hour allocated for this task, so I stated firmly that she must stop, adding that if she couldn't listen to me because she was so angry with me and angry at everything, I'd have to put the paints away for today. Diane was still unable to control herself and I had to put the paints away, acknowledging at the same time that Diane was very angry with me.

> D: [suddenly subdued as I shut the cupboard on the paints] Okay, then, I'll help clean up.
> V: [surprised tone] That's quick! I thought you'd take a while to get over being so angry with me. You want to help now?

Instead, Diane darted over suddenly to the toy hammer, then picked up the baby doll (male) she had earlier placed in her den.

> D: [to the doll] It's *you* I hate.
> V: You're not saying you hate me now. You want to get at the doll.

She forcefully began to beat at the doll's eyes and mouth with the hammer (not inflicting any real damage on the doll) and repeatedly calling it horrible. Making as if to destroy it, she raised the hammer again and again chanting 'I want to *hurt* you, I want to hurt you, I want to hurt you'.

> V: [as Diane continued beating the doll] Very angry, first with me. Now you're angry with the little one . . . wanting to hurt it.

Diane turned to the basin, put in the plug, and ran the water full force over the doll's face, as I said the doll couldn't get away, couldn't breathe. Tossing it face down into the water, Diane ended with: 'Now mum won't have a son.'

> V: You hurt him. That way you hurt your Mum.

Diane paused, went limp, and sat down. I said, 'You're tired from all that anger and hurting. I'll start cleaning the room up now.'

Diane sat very still and watched me for a while, then decided to clean the doll herself. She shampooed the doll's hair, pretending to make certain the soap didn't sting its eyes, then carefully wrapped it up. She asked anxiously whether the doll would be safe where she had left it to dry, 'because it may explode.' I reassured her that it would be safe until her next session and that she hadn't harmed the doll in any way, even though she'd felt so angry with it. 'I would have stopped you before anything was hurt or broken.'

In her next (eleventh) session, Diane took up the doll immediately, then changed the role-play after quick deliberation: 'I want to play something different. Mums. I'm the Mum and you're the daughter.' We worked at jobs around the house together, and became excited because we planned to go to the beach later. At the beach the daughter was surprised because she was sent off on her own to play, but went happily, only to return to her mother and find that she had vanished. Devastated, the daughter eventually reached home on her own, after looking everywhere for her mother. When her mother opened the door, the daughter accused her mother angrily of leaving her. The mother coolly answered 'Sorry.' The daughter became even more angry at this response.

Unexpectedly, the mother in turn became very angry with her daughter. She commanded her to dress the baby, but the daughter defiantly refused. This provoked the mother into an even greater rage, although by now the daughter had become frightened and tried to placate her. The mother came towards the daughter menacingly and put deep red gouges down the daughter's cheek, taking her time with a slow, calculated action. (Diane deliberately pressed her finger down my cheek, hard enough to leave a red mark, but not enough to hurt.) The daughter, numbed with shock, looked in the mirror and became even more frightened. She had to pretend she felt calm and pleasant to her mother, even though being deeply affected. It was a terrible blow to think that her own mother had wounded her and to realize, too, that other people would know when they saw her face.

The daughter tried hard to be good, but the mother, although now unprovoked, shouted at her to stop talking. She beat the daughter on the head with her fists (in practice, only lightly). The daughter cried and said 'ow, ow' very softly, holding her cheeks and head.

D: Work now!
V: Can I go, Mum? Can I go now?
D: Yes. No. Come back here. Give me that tie. (V. does everything to please her, robot-like).
D: Thank you. You may go.

Diane suddenly transformed herself into a kind mother who returned from work, saw the daughter's face and gently cleaned her wounds, saying in a solicitous voice, 'What's the matter, my dear? My dear, my dear [shaking her head from side to side]. What's the matter? Please tell me what's the matter'. Although the daughter at first couldn't believe the injuries would heal, they did eventually. She was grateful for the kindness, but became confused about the identity of her mother. The kind Mum explained that the other woman was mean and had fooled the daughter into believing she could be trusted.

The second mum then bought the girl a special toy and the girl enjoyed playing with it, but this Mum kept offering her more, more toys than she could possibly play with. So the girl tried to stop this Mum from giving her too much by refusing things, but she noticed the Mum's feelings were then hurt. The girl reacted by trying to play more frantically with all the toys (with Diane directing me to say to her that the last one was my 'special favourite' toy). This response made the Mum encourage the girl to play even more and the girl played strenuously, trying to please the Mum.

Diane, who had directed all the action in the story as she always did, had us quickly switch roles at this point. She became the older sister and I was the younger brother again. As brother and sister, we enjoyed playing with all the new toys, but then we started thinking neither of us had enough. We fought over who got more, ending up at the sand box fighting over the sand toys. Diane now started splatting sand on the floor, saying over and over: 'It's mine! It's mine!'

V: You want more. And you're looking at the clock, maybe wanting more time here, too. Not easy to leave when you don't want to. But it's time to leave now.
D: Before everything gets covered in sand.
V: [laughing] Yes, we don't have extra time today to tidy up.

Diane laughed too and ran to her foster carer, who was surprised to be given a quick hug.

Diane immediately returned to the sand box in her next session, placing herself in the role of kind mum and me in the role of the girl. I enjoyed having her care for me while my parents were gone but this mum then learned that my parents had disappeared for good. She was very kind to me and told me the news gently, while I enacted reactions of disbelief and protest, following Diane's directions. The new mum took care of the girl, but tired eventually of her crying and complaints, accusing the girl of not caring for her as a mum. The girl then tried to become more cheerful, realising that she was worried when her new mum's feelings were hurt. She needed this mum to look after her, even though she still loved her Mum and Dad.

Diane's serious mood abruptly changed and she playfully threw the playdough across the room to me, inviting me to join in. I did, saying as we played and relaxed that she wanted to have fun now, to make herself change from being so worried and sad. At the end I told her that we had three more sessions together (since funding had run out for good now, although I had recommended a further ten sessions, to stabilize Diane's progress).

Discussion of the second phase of Diane's play therapy

From the sixth session onwards, Diane's activity in play therapy became emotionally much deeper and more powerful, and she seemed to have altered significantly both in her attitude towards herself and in her physical appearance. That she herself was able to choose whether or not to continue with the play therapy seems to have been a significant factor in this change. Non-directive play therapy, by building into the therapeutic contract the child's choice jointly with the therapist's for more sessions, enabled Diane to redress her experiences of helplessness which were likely to have arisen from adult over-control, during her physically and emotionally abusive experiences, and during her removal from home to foster care. The choice of more sessions also gave her the opportunity to exercise control over an event in her current life and to express a need at a time when, because of the long delay in court proceedings, her future care was indeterminate and potentially frightening to her.

Yet because at least some of her emotional needs were being addressed in her sessions, Diane seemed to feel more confident, hid her face less, sought out new experiences and began to make herself up as a more true-to-life character than in her earlier sessions. However, she still initially kept the structure of events the same, trying out her new appearance within a safely established routine, dressing up as an Indian, but then applying more realistic make-up rather than Indian warpaint. At the beginning of the later session, when she made herself up as a proud, mean witch, her increased confidence meant that she could start acting out fully the negative role which she had touched on earlier, but had swiftly rejected, presumably as being too threatening.

The earlier theme of messiness also re-emerged and was equated with naughtiness, but was addressed in a rather more personal way, with Diane herself having a messy face, for which she is chastised. Her attitude towards her physical self, her sense of wishing to be different and more colourful was also expressed in her dressing up and her dancing and physical movement, which became freer and more exuberant as the sessions progressed. Through the elaborate role-plays, which we shall analyse more fully later, Diane addressed the ambivalent feelings involved for her in her relationship with her brother, and, most intensely of all, her feelings of anger, powerless and revenge, as well as a deep sense of bereavement and continuing love towards her mother. In the role play, Diane then was able to focus on her feelings of bereavement for her parents, and the growing attachment between herself and her foster carer. Her throwing game at the end of this session seemed to be a prelude to her last three sessions, where she seemed to be using play predominantly to work out her current concerns and feelings.

Diane's final sessions

Diane entered the room for her next session, saying she had lots more playing to do and wanting more sessions. I had to tell her that we had three more times left, because there was no more money for my work. I knew she wanted more and was disappointed. With her head down, Diane looked through the dressing up box, remembering the Indian costume that she had worn at the beginning, and involving me in a brief dance round the room, playing music on the trumpet. (I commented: 'Remembering all the things you like to do here.') She then went to the sand box, assigning me the little brother, and herself the big sister, role. Flicking the sand out of the sand box, Diane instigated a sand fight with her little brother. She became very excited, throwing sand around the area of the sand box and making sure that I participated. (I had several times to remind her not to throw sand too near my eyes.) The sand was emptied eventually onto the floor; Diane took her shoes off and stomped in the sand, chanting. I said, 'That's a good mess', and Diane agreed, 'Great isn't it. Let's wash our hands and feet now so we can go on the carpet.' As we washed together, we talked easily about stopping ten minutes early today to tidy up.

The scene changed quickly after this. Diane put on a black cloak, and changed into a Mum who was in a bad mood, bossing her daughter around and taking all her pretty things away from her. The daughter felt frightened of her Mum, of what she'd do to her, and take from her. The daughter also felt ugly, as if she would never have anything pretty to keep, never have anything at all she liked.

Diane abruptly stopped at this point, turned away from me, and painted silently at the far end of the room for the last ten minutes. She carefully mixed her own colours and painted two pictures of brightly coloured flowers, bringing them out to give to her foster carer for the new bulletin board in their kitchen.

Diane began the following session by playing in the sand with me as her younger brother, kindly showing him how to play and also letting him imitate her actions. But she became tired of his constant company and wanted time with her own friends. She went to phone a friend, and then got cross with her brother for listening, saying that 'little boys' shouldn't listen to private conversations. The friend helped her play a trick on 'the nuisance', by taking him to the park and then leaving him there. (In my role as little brother, I wasn't supposed to hear this, but it was a good way of keeping me informed of the plot.) The younger brother was rescued later and seemed confused about what had happened to him, but then became deeply distressed when he trustingly went back to the park with his sister and her friends and everyone hid from him. The brother became angry with his sister when he discovered their trick. Diane then ran and got the doll and made as if to bite its finger off. I said, 'Don't really do that – it will break', and Diane took a felt tip pen, drawing red gashes with felt tips on the doll from his neck to his stomach. I commented on her anger as she worked, but Diane stopped abruptly when I said. 'The little one is hurt – everyone can see how hurt it is now.'

She shifted to mixing paints and ended the session with a messy game of catch on her own.

Diane's last session began with her holding her left arm cradled in her right hand, in a quite exaggerated manner. She explained that she had hurt herself running up the stairs. She then began making a paint mixture on her own, sending me (still in my role of little brother) to the opposite end of the room to draw. After a long interval, I was allowed to help her as she experimented adding different amounts of colour to her mixture. When she was satisfied with the result she washed her hands, and looked at the mixture with pleasure. She swirled the colours and they separated out repeatedly into new but different combinations.

Diane then suggested that we draw a big picture of a flower garden together. Following her lead, we decorated the border and printed our names along the outside. We talked about leaving, Diane saying she wanted to come again: 'You'll *have* to see me if I come and see you.' I acknowledged that she wanted to come back. I added that I wished we had more time together too, and that I also hoped that she would not have any more big problems in the future. Diane quickly returned to our painting looking momentarily threatened. As she left, she looked into the sink, smiled and nodded to herself. My last comment was that the mixture she made changes and gets better every time she looks at it. When I myself came to leave, I found a letter from her in the waiting room: 'Dear Virginia, Thank you for playing games. I had a good time with you. I don't no how to thank you for having me. P.S. No Painting and Stiring With Out me.'

Discussion of the final phase of Diane's therapy

In order to prepare Diane for ending her sessions, the therapist mentioned to Diane at the beginning of the thirteenth session that there were three sessions left, acknowledging as she did so Diane's reluctance about ending. In her play at the beginning of this session, Diane recapitulated some of the themes of her early sessions, such as dressing up and playing music, as she seemed to come to terms with leaving. Her current relationship with her brother was addressed in the next play sequence, with a sand fight between herself and the therapist (as her little brother). The therapist was still needed by Diane for help in controlling her intense feelings and actions while play-fighting and making a mess. But Diane was very satisfied with the outcome and could take genuine and spontaneous pleasure in actively making a mess. She demonstrated her ability to set limits on her own messiness herself when she cleaned her own hands and feet.

In her last session, Diane was able to work cooperatively with the therapist and discuss most of her strong feelings about their ending directly. It was however difficult for both the therapist and Diane to finish, even though it had been planned for, because of the therapist's sense of 'unfinished business' and Diane's continuing message of it 'not being enough'. (We discuss Diane's ending further in the next section on practice issues.)

Diane again played out painful feelings about previous experiences with her mother, acting out the deep emotional damage she had suffered from her, which had left her with a recurring sense of fear at her mother's anger and a sense of ugliness which seemed to stem from her mother's abusive care. By painting flower pictures for her foster carers' kitchen, she seemed to be finding a means of restoring her sense of self-worth through creating an attractive environment for herself, as well as for others, and seemed to be acknowledging to herself that the foster carer was responding with respect to her.

In the last role-play where she tricked her brother, her current mixed feelings towards him were expressed, showing both her feelings of kindliness and helpfulness towards him, but also her feelings of anger and restriction from his dependency on her. As well as showing Diane's own personally vital coping mechanism of displacement of anger towards a powerful adult on to a less threatening child, her role-plays also suggest a possible more general mechanism for the inter-generational transmission of abuse. In her last session, Diane seemed to be continuing her therapeutic progress and used appropriate symbolic means, including verbal messages to work through her varied feelings about ending.

PRACTICE ISSUES

Role-playing within non-directive play therapy

Role-play and pretending, as Irwin (1983) points out, have been at the heart of many forms of treatment, such as psychodrama, gestalt therapy and certain forms of behaviour therapy. They have been widely used with adults as well as children.

In non-directive play therapy, because the child chooses the means to express herself, she can try out a wide range of possible activities symbolising her experiences, feelings and emotional difficulties, and discover, as Diane did in role-play, the vehicle that best suits her needs.

The advantage of this non-directive approach is that it not only allows the child to find the activity with the best emotional 'fit', but also to use such an activity when she is ready to do so. Thus with Diane, it is possible to see her early dressing up and dance routines as the beginnings of her discovery of the right 'form'; she also embarked on these symbolically charged and complex enactments when she was ready to do so. The timing of this appeared to be significant. The therapist had, we would guess, shown herself to be trustworthy (for example, in the fifth session by recognising and acknowledging Diane's feelings of discomfiture and the source of Diane's misunderstandings about play therapy). Even more importantly, perhaps, Diane at this point was assured of there being time enough, with more sessions available, to explore a deeper level of her experience through the play therapy sessions. She seemed to have greater confidence in herself, the therapist, the approach, and the rules of the playroom environment itself. Because some of her urgent needs were now being recognised, she was able to play with greater fluidity and in a less inhibited way than was seen, for example, in her earlier tentative attempts at exploratory play with the finger paints. Finally, the choice of form seems significant; Diane had already been showing her wish to find a means of expressing herself which would adequately reflect the stronger feelings that she had hitherto felt too constrained to reveal.

There are several practice points to consider in helping the child within a role-play. The first is a more general one concerning the support that needs to be available for the child outside the sessions, which Diane's sessions illustrate. For example, before the role-play depicting herself and her brother, she made a card for her foster mother, and then gave this to her at the end of the enactment. Her seeking out of reassurance underlines the importance for children of having adequate parenting and support while addressing early emotionally damaging experiences. The therapist cannot and must not be the child's sole emotional support. (See Wilson, 1993, and Chapter 5 for a further discussion.)

Other issues for the therapist in role-plays relate particularly to how much she adds to or fleshes out the role given to her by the child, in what ways she elucidates the child's feelings within the role-play, and whether or not to depart at any point from the directives given by the child. The underlying principles of non-directive play therapy, that the therapist reflects the child's feelings, is helpful up to a point, but does not give specific guidance on these more complex questions.

Often a child of Diane's age starts, as she did, by giving the therapist some instruction about what to do or say. (See Ben's last session, chapter 7, for another example.) The therapist is then conforming to a normal 'metacommunication' device within symbolic play; such devices begin to be utilized by children, as we discussed in Patrick's chapter, from a young age.

Of course, children sometimes enact role plays in which they themselves take all the parts, as we see Ben doing in chapter 7. Under these circumstances the therapist's usual role, as it was with Diane as an Indian, is one of an observer and/or admirer ('the audience'), or one of a narrator of the character's actions and commentator on the actor's thoughts and feelings. In fact, even when the child deliberately excludes the therapist, say by an instruction to turn away and 'not to look' during a play sequence, perhaps signalling independence from or discomfort with the therapist's direct attention, the child still on some level seems to remain alert to the therapist. The child's responses seem adapted to the belief that the therapist remains interested and available for further communication when the child so chooses. In this sense the therapist can still be viewed as the child's (passive) audience.

When the therapist is directly or indirectly invited to participate in a roleplay, she needs to have developed sufficient acting skills to respond in role. At the same time, care needs to be taken about acting the part *too* realistically, especially with younger or traumatised children, since this may frighten and confuse them; with older children it may distract them from their own play. And at the beginning of the enactment in particular the therapist needs to check with the child on how to behave. For instance, when Diane told the therapist to say, 'I'm not frightened', the therapist repeated it. Noticing that Diane by contrast was acting frightened, the therapist commented on this and then asked, *sotto voce*, 'Are you still pretending to be scared?', before saying aloud, 'She's scared and

I'm not'. The critical shifts in the role-plays emanated in this manner from Diane herself. Thus, in this particular role-play, Diane introduced the idea that she was the Black Witch, that she had put a spell on her mother, that the mother, as the victim, was lying and so on.

However, the therapist may choose at certain points to add to her role, without having specific directions from the child. Thus, when the mother's wickedness had been discovered by Diane, who felt deeply betrayed by her, the therapist in the mother's role realised that, in this situation, she would naturally feel terribly guilty and ashamed of herself. Guided by these feelings, the therapist enacted feelings of deep shame for the evil that she had done to Diane. At this point, it seemed to the therapist highly unlikely that Diane's mother would have expressed these emotions to Diane. Nor did Diane herself give such an instruction within the role-play. But in non-directive play therapy, as well as taking directions from the child, the therapist may use her own feeling in an emotionally healthy way. The role-play then becomes a *symbolic* means of restoring relationships and as such may have deep significance for the child. Diane's feelings were deeply involved in this enactment, as her expressive language shows:

> D: [with anguish] You tricked me. How could you trick me?
> V: [in a loud voice] I didn't think you'd ever find out. You were just a little girl, I thought, and I could do what I wanted.
> D: [deeply offended] I'm not just a little girl.
> V: You mean, you could understand? Now I feel so awful [choked voice] about it because I didn't ever want you to know I did bad things. I wanted you to think I was always good . . . I didn't want you to grow up and find out I did bad things.
> D: [in brighter tone] Well, I forgive you.
> V: [hopeful, then dejected] Do you? I don't see how you could, they were so wicked.
> D: [alert voice] Here's a trumpet. I'll play with you. It might cheer you up . . . I just wanted to get back at you for telling me to clean all that mess off my face . . .

Diane thus seemed able, using a wide range of emotions, symbolically to work towards forgiving her mother, and explaining and justifying her actions. The therapist responded to this with the following comment: 'So really it was the only way you could tell me that you were angry with me. You had to get back at me in such a bad way and then you found out everything.'

The therapist was helping Diane to 'name and own' the anger she felt towards her mother in the role-play. This sequence also demonstrates one of the key strengths of psychodrama as a therapeutic technique: the role-play allows the actor to experience intense, 'real' emotions. However, because it is a 'play', these emotions are safer to express, being at one step removed from reality. Enacting these emotions in actuality might have caused Diane severe anxiety; it was fraught with the potentially realistic danger of a very hurtful, rejecting response from her mother. Ben's role-play in chapter 7 about his father has similar features; both children portray deep-seated 'wish fulfilments', resolving the abusive relationships they had experienced with their parents in a more positive way.

Abuser/child role-plays

A prominent feature of both these children's role-plays, as in many other role-plays by abused children, is that the child takes on the abuser's role. As a child's overall development advances, these role-plays often move from very rudimentary child-abuser roles to more complex combinations and shifts in roles within the role-play itself, as Diane's sessions illustrate. Role-plays in which the child takes the abuser's role serve the emotional and cognitive functions of allowing a previously powerless, abused child to redress his or her negative experience and become powerful in play, thus adjusting this previously 'unjust' and 'unnatural' adult/child relationship. The child is also able to experience personally the child's role from an outside perspective. As part of this perspective the child is likely to realise more clearly what his or her own feelings and responses were. She or he may also recognise that another person (the therapist in the child's role) has a deep enough understanding of these earlier experiences to be able to play them out with emotional accuracy and sensitivity. Finally, the child in the abuser's role is simultaneously acting out the abuser's feelings and actions, and is enabled to develop a greater understanding of the abusing adult's behaviour, all of which Diane demonstrates vividly in the above role-play sequence (see Wilson and Ryan, 1994a).

There are, however, certain unresolved issues surrounding the practice of role-plays of abusive situations with children who have been emotionally damaged by these kinds of experiences. One is whether the therapist should give normalising, 'moral' responses to the child who is playing the abuser's role. By participating in the destruction of the abusing parent, for example, does the therapist tacitly condone violent solutions and retributions? Should the therapist make 'normalising' responses such as 'We can pretend to hurt others in here, but we can't *really*'? The therapist must give serious thought to these issues and attempt to satisfy herself that the child does clearly understand the differences between both pretence and reality and moral judgements of right and wrong, as Diane clearly seemed to.

In cases where the child shows reality/fantasy confusions or has not developed a basic encoding of moral constraints (see chapter 5), the therapist needs to make direct, clear statements on these specific features of the child's role-plays. (Some other therapists, however, may wish to address this issue more directly at the beginning of their work with a child.)

Another problematic practice issue surrounding role-plays with abuser/child roles is whether the abused child suffers additional emotional harm if he or she chooses to play the role of the abused child, and assigns the therapist the abuser's role (Carroll, 1994). Again, a clinical judgement is needed on whether the child understands and enacts the abused role on the level of pretence, rather than being completely immersed in the victim's role. It also seems necessary in these (rarer) cases, for the therapist in the abuser's role to give her normalising responses (e.g. 'almost all adults would stop themselves and know this is very wrong'). In other words, here, as in other role-plays, the therapist has a vital role in enabling the child to hold together 'reality' and 'play', thus ensuring that the child does not become lost or confused in the feelings experienced in role. This issue lies within the domain of drama therapy and seems to be akin to that described by professional stage actors, who are careful not to become so identified with the part they are playing that they lose their sense of performing and being 'in role'.

It is also important in these cases, as in all other role-plays, that the therapist direct the child to symbolic re-enactments of abuse involving socially and personally acceptable, and safe areas of the therapist's and child's bodies. This may include prohibiting bodily damage and destruction of materials as the therapist did with Diane. (See also chapters on Delroy and Patricia.)

Finally, in our experience with abused children, the child usually places the therapist in the abuser's role when the child intends to vanquish the adult and in fantasy become a powerful child-avenger, as Diane did (and see Chapter 7). This intent may be a necessary step for a child in working through abusive experiences towards healthier functioning. (See Pynoos and Eth, 1986, for a discussion of the role of fantasy fulfilments in the resolution of emotionally harmful experiences by severely traumatised children).

Role-play and interpretation

In our earlier book, we suggest that there is sometimes a fine line between reflection and interpretation. In responding during Diane's role-plays within the role assigned to her, the therapist also, at times, clarified for Diane some of the feelings which she was experiencing. Although speaking in role, the therapist was thus 'explaining' or interpreting in a very basic sense Diane's feelings to her. However, with a non-directive approach, beyond this basic sense of interpretation, the therapist accepts the child's choice of symbolic activity and responds within the metaphor used by the child, without interpretation.

As we discussed earlier the therapist formed hypotheses *to herself* about the meaning of Diane's play, in order to understand and respond to it better, but these explanations were never shared with Diane. Instead, the therapist used her inner hypothesising and own feelings congruently to help Diane from within the metaphor of her play.

Diane's responses in one role play in particular suggested that she had only incompletely worked through her difficulties surrounding her relationship with her brother. Thus in her penultimate session, when she put red lines down the doll's body and the therapist commented that she wanted to hurt it and was very angry with it, Diane stopped abruptly and turned to mixing paints. Although a reflection rather than an interpretation, the therapist's verbalisation of Diane's feelings of anger and desire to harm the doll seemed extremely threatening to her, and was possibly too direct a reflection of feelings which were still difficult to acknowledge. Diane's move away from the dolls to the playdough was accepted readily by the therapist, and illustrates one way in which the non-directive approach accepts a child's retention of needed defensive responses.

Evaluating therapeutic progress

In our next chapter (Anna) we consider the therapist's reasoning in deciding to end Anna's sessions when she did. It is evident in Diane's story, as with those of most of the other children in this book, that children within the local authority care system usually have many more complex and protracted life decisions weighing on them than Anna did. This makes working with them in the first place (as we describe in our story of Delroy) and completing therapeutic work with them more difficult.

As we have suggested elsewhere (Ryan and Wilson, 1995b), a therapist formulates working hypotheses throughout therapeutic work with a child. An integral part of this task is evaluating therapeutic progress along key dimensions. These key dimensions incorporate normal and abnormal developmental theory and research, informing the therapist's judgment of whether the child is making progress towards having a normal developmental trajectory activated or restored. These key dimensions are also child-specific: that is the therapist also selects out the particular child's resiliences and weaknesses from the many available during any child's development, which the therapist then attunes to more carefully.

For the therapist working with Diane and other children involved in care proceedings, whose futures are undecided, one key dimension is often anxiety: to what extent does the basic anxiety which a child normally feels over a precarious future – and sometimes a precarious immediate future – contribute to his or her anxiety within sessions, to abnormally anxious responses outside sessions, and to impediments to any therapeutic progress. Given each child's unique position, added to the overall complexity of many of these cases, no automatic 'rule of thumb' can be applied. However, Diane's story does provide clues to guide judgements of a child's progress and to generate hypotheses for conducting sorely needed outcome research on therapeutic work with children in statutory settings.

First of all, Diane noticeably chose to avoid talking about or playing out any future for herself within her sessions. Her avoidance of the topic, followed by her role-plays of past and current worries and distressing emotions, seemed to indicate that Diane's concern about her future was high. It could potentially be pervading all her inner life and outer responses, and became an urgent recommendation for permanency in the therapist's assessment of Diane for the court. If funding constraints had not curtailed their work, the therapist, working along with Diane's social worker and foster carer, might perhaps have helped Diane to address this issue if she so chose, during later sessions, although real uncertainty about her future might even so have impeded this therapeutic help. This concern and others outlined below, were stated to the court and to the local authority in the therapist's final report when her involvement ended.

One further emotional issue seemed unresolved at the conclusion of Diane's therapy. She needed more help, in the therapist's opinion, in finding more appropriate expressions of her feelings and responses when she became angry, most particularly when this was with a person whom she loved and with whom she had a dependent relationship or who was dependent on her. The therapist also found it noteworthy that Diane had not addressed the other significant relationship for most children, that with her father, in any detail. Nor did the therapist have any evidence as to why this should be so, other than general hypotheses, such as Diane's emotional overload with other significant relationships and changes which precluded her emotional capacity to address this relationship.

The therapist recognised at the same time that Diane made considerable progress in her resolution of deep emotional pain and distress concerning her mother and her mother's abuse of her. Diane also was able to show her growing attachment to and dependency on her foster carer, both of which were emotionally healthy, recent developments. Other signs of identifiable progress by the end of her play therapy sessions were her age-appropriate behaviour in mixing colours rather than making a mess, her changed and more confident attitude towards herself, and her co-operative behaviour in the play therapy sessions. This was reflected in her behaviour at school and in the foster home, where she was reported to be more responsive, sociable and communicative.

In evaluating Diane's progress in therapy, then, the therapist took account of changes in her behaviour and in the themes of her activities in the sessions, as well as evidence of reported changes in other key areas of her life. Certain issues remained unresolved, in the therapist's opinion because of the premature curtailment of Diane's therapy and her unresolved care plan.

THEORETICAL ISSUE

Physical abuse and play therapy

The main issue to be explored here concerns the impact that the experience of physical abuse can have on the individual child. Recent preoccupation with sexual abuse has led to a relative neglect in theory and in practice of the negative psychological impact that physical abuse may have on a child. Although it has long been recognised that physical abuse can be the visible sign of other forms of maltreatment, which need to be addressed therapeutically, there sometimes appears to be a tacit assumption with children who have suffered predominantly physical abuse that, provided they are physically safe and are beginning to feel secure, little long-term psychological damage will result from the injury. In our practice experience, for example, it is much easier to secure funding for therapy for children who have experienced sexual abuse rather than those who have been physically or emotionally abused. However, in the work with Diane and from Diane's behaviour at the time of referral it was quite clear that, although she had lived for a year with sympathetic and supportive foster carers, the emotional damage of her earlier experiences still remained, and continued to affect her current behaviour. Of course, as we suggest above, it seems highly probable that her difficulties were compounded by the continued uncertainties about what her future would be. Nonetheless, her current behaviour in her foster home and at school, as well as the issues which emerged in her play, suggested that many of her continuing problems were the result of her traumatic and unresolved relationships with her birth family. Diane's sessions demonstrate that physical abuse leaves psychological as well as physical scars. This psychological impact is supported by research which suggests that the 'difficult' personality characteristics of some infants and children may be the result of repeated abusive or neglectful behaviours on the part of their principal carers (Crittenden, 1985). These attachment issues are now being recognized within a broad developmental psychopathology model of child maltreatment. This model is only now beginning to influence therapeutic interventions with both the child and caregivers (Cicchetti, 1989).

However, much of the earlier research evidence on the short- and long-term consequences of physical abuse – in itself surprisingly scanty at least in comparison to that on sexual abuse – offered what can appear to be a very undifferentiated account of its impact. Martin and Beezley (1977), for example, listed nine characteristics derived from their research, ranging from impaired ability for enjoyment to hypervigilance, which they found in varying proportions in physically abused children. We consider these in more detail below but the limitations of their usefulness for those working with abused children are obvious; the list reads like a comprehensive account of social-emotional disorders in children. It is not necessarily useful, then, in helping us to identify the specific impact physical abuse may have on an individual child. Furthermore, this list cannot make the necessary links between the abusive experience itself and the particular problems revealed by the child. We want to show here how some of the rather bald characteristics identified in this type of research on children's physical abuse manifested themselves in Diane's play and behaviour, and began to be resolved in her play therapy.

First, we shall discuss how we relate the child's experience of physical abuse to a child's mental development, using the framework set out in the Introduction and in our earlier book. In this explanation, we have broadly followed Piaget's conceptualisation of the child's development of mental structures, because it seems useful to describe experiences as involving responses at three different levels of functioning: the emotional, feeling level; the cognitive, intellectual level; *and* the motor or physical level.

Briefly, a child's experience can be conceptualised as being assimilated and accommodating itself to pre-existing mental schemas. In the course of normal development, children will have developed (and be developing) relatively permanent affective schemas towards their carers. These incorporate strong positive feelings towards carers and, although negative affect will also be experienced towards the caregivers, the balance of a child's feelings will be positive rather than negative (Erikson, 1963). [Attachment theorists' descriptions of children's internal working models are closely related to this conceptualisation – see Bowlby (1979)]. Cicchetti describes these working models as 'constructed out of the children's own actions, the feedback they receive from these actions and the actions of caregivers . . . there will be wide variations across individuals in working models, and individuals' working models will fairly accurately reflect their own experience as well as cognitive, linguistic and behavioural skills. These internal working models, once organised, tend to operate outside conscious awareness and resist dramatic change' (1989: 398).

With physically abusive experiences, strong negative feelings (anger, hatred, fear) are aroused in the child. The child has great difficulty in accommodating these powerful negative experiences to his or her already existing, relatively permanent affective schemas. Strong polarised feelings are in direct conflict with one another and hinder the child's development just because they are so difficult to resolve. The child will largely be unable to integrate schemas of 'good' parent and 'bad' parent into higher level, more advanced and flexible schemas, thus making these conflicting affective schemas less mobile, less conscious and less well-integrated than those of a non-abused child.

We are all of us, of course, to some extent 'stuck' with our early experiences, or within the framework adopted here, the schemas that result from them. However, the immobility resulting from the difficulty of reconciling positive with extremely negative experiences explains, for example, why an emotionally damaged person is so much more likely to form a pattern of repeated damaging relationships in later life. It also explains why the effects of cumulative experience of abuse, and faulty attachments, coupled with other determinants such as poverty, social isolation, stress and more general familial violence (Kaufman and Zigler, 1989), can make it difficult for abused children's internal structures to change without direct intervention (Cicchetti, 1989). A history of physical abuse can also lead into abusive parenting experiences of the next generation of children, discussed further below. (The extent of intergenerational transmission of abuse is estimated by Kaufman and Zigler to be approximately one-third of known physically abusive incidents.)

Conflicts also coexist for a child on a physical, or motor, level. Since physical abuse necessarily involves parts of the body, a child will have difficulty assimilating abusive bodily sensations and responses (e.g. disfigurement, pain or withdrawal) and accommodating these experiences to existing mental schemas associated, say, with physical care, exploration of the environment or physical expression of affection. (Such conflicting motor behaviours are, for example, the carer hugging the child at one time but violently pushing the child away at another, or the carer washing the child's face one minute and slapping it in anger the next.) Repeated abusive experiences, or even a single severely traumatic one, may lead a child to develop strong negative motor responses, such as Diane's messiness, affective responses such as her passivity and aggressiveness, and negative bodily schemas, such as her sense of ugliness and disfigurement.

Physical abuse engenders extreme conflict on a cognitive level as well, because a child experiences great mental confusion about a carer who is both responsible for, but simultaneously harms, him or her. This mental confusion may be actively and consciously experienced or a child may develop relatively permanent and logical explanations to resolve this extreme discrepancy cognitively (e.g. 'I am unlovable, therefore my father beats me', or 'I am ugly, therefore my mother kicks me').

These conflicts begin to explain why patterns of behaviour which are identified in the research on physical abuse as characteristic of the physically abused child can appear to be so opposite, for example, physically abused children are said to manifest consistently higher levels of aggression, but also often appear passive and withdrawn. We shall now summarise these research findings, and then show how they appeared in Diane's behaviour and in her play therapy.

The literature generally recognises that, as a consequence of physical abuse, a child tends to make unhealthy emotional adaptations in order to survive in this abusive environment. Four major personality traits are consistently seen in the physically abused child: passivity, aggressiveness, regression and interpersonal relationship difficulties. We consider these briefly in turn.

Passivity is often cited in this research literature (e.g. Muir, 1976) as a major distinguishing feature of the abused child. The child's behaviour may be characterised by frozen watchfulness (first described thus by Ounsted et al., 1974), lack of initiative, hypervigilance and pseudo-adult behaviours.

'Frozen watchfulness' is seen as a child's attempt to cope with the caregiver's unpredictable behaviour, where basic trust and a secure environment have not been established. Older children may become extremely passive and withdrawn, show little initiative, avoid attracting attention to themselves, and typically do not act until they are fairly certain of the adult reaction. The child may become hypervigilant, be acutely sensitive to adult mood changes and concentrate all resources on his or her caregivers in order to please them and avoid further harm. Since children are only appreciated when they meet adult needs, they often take on pseudo-adult behaviours that result in a role-reversal between child and parent. Because so much is being invested emotionally in this relationship and also because to do so may be hazardous, the child plays little, does not explore the environment and does not develop peer relationships outside the family.

The behaviour of the physically abused child may also show marked *aggression* and be characterised by anger and violence, social ineptness, poor impulse control, delinquency, self-hatred and passive–aggressive behaviour. Severe physical punishment has been associated with a lowering of the aggressive threshold, and appears to be a major factor in the development of a range of deviant behaviours. Provocative and overactive behaviour may be adopted, seemingly to attract attention, albeit abusive attention, from unresponsive adults, or as a means of testing out new relationships, thus reinforcing a negative self-image, or to allay the extreme anxiety involved in anticipating physical injury by ensuring that it occurs sooner, and is under the child's control, in the sense that the child seeks to have it over and done with.

The abused child may also show *regression*, characterised by enuresis, day-dreaming, masturbation or nightmares. Some children regress to earlier behaviours in order to cope with an abusive environment, often paradoxically becoming overly dependent while at the same time withdrawing from even positive adult attention. Their helplessness is exaggerated, seemingly in an attempt to gain sympathy and thus avoid injury. They may also develop abnormal and/or self-stimulatory behaviours to cope with abuse.

Finally, the abused child may often experience *interpersonal relationship deficits*, involving a poor self-concept, low self-esteem, lack of autonomy, poor social skills, social isolation and loneliness. The inconsistency of the abusive environment prevents the development of trust, the establishment of a sense of self-worth, and hence a sure base from which to develop satisfying relationships with others. Although this is rarely touched on in the literature, our clinical experience, as Diane illustrates, also suggests that, at a conscious level, embarrassment about physical injuries and, at a deeper level, a sense of physical impairment, may also prevent the child from developing a sense of bodily attractiveness and wholeness.

The two personality traits of passivity and aggression can be seen to develop partly as the consequence of a curtailment of normal exploratory behaviour, which in turn has resulted from the need to be extremely careful over how to behave at home. The anxiety surrounding this need to be careful and indeed unobtrusive also means that the child cannot develop an internalised sense of what is or is not appropriate by way of exploratory behaviour.

In Diane's case, the description of her at the time of referral as passive, but also intermittently aggressive towards her younger brother and other children, had the hallmarks of a child who has been abused and suggested that she had developed these responses as a result of the uncertainties of her home life. In play therapy, as well as wishing to be seen as 'good' by the therapist, these impulses appeared as a preoccupation with tidiness and messiness, which are often associated, especially for girls, with being good and being naughty.

These concerns emerged, as we have seen, as a theme in Diane's play, which she addressed first through tentative experimentation with paints, and then, as she grew more confident, through intensely messy play. Two points seem to have particular significance here. First, the play therapist's reassurance, after Diane had personalised the balloon, that no one would get hurt by it. Second, the help given by the play therapist not only in accepting the messy activity but also in setting a limit on Diane's behaviour (making sure that she got clean before moving out of that area of the playroom), which enabled Diane to experience, and then begin to internalise for herself, controls on exploratory behaviour. As Case (1990) comments, messiness may symbolise power and danger simultaneously: Diane clearly found this messiness both exhilarating and disturbing, as she must have done in her earlier experiences at home. She felt powerful in making the mess and in controlling the balloon, but needed the therapist to reassure her and to set firm limits on her behaviour, thereby beginning to remove the strong sense of danger and threat involved in the act of being messy.

By the conclusion of her therapy – and it is interesting that she chose to return to this painting activity towards the end – it seemed that Diane had resolved many of these issues. Her activity showed an age-appropriate level of exploration, so that she spent time making a mixture, using paint and other materials in a deliberate, concentrated and organised way, and watched with pleasure as the mixture changed colour.

The personality traits of passivity and difficulties in relationships with others are also evident in Diane's attitude towards her physical self and in her self-concept. The need to be unobtrusive in order to avoid further abuse, which contributes, as we have seen, to the passivity and withdrawn behaviour of a physically abused child, also undermines the child's sense of self-worth, since the parental response suggests that the child is only valued, or at least tolerated, if inconspicuous.

These patterns of adaptation to abuse emerged quickly as important therapeutic issues with Diane's dressing up, her music and video, and painting her face in striking colours. We would hypothesise from this behaviour that Diane had strong feelings, which she was unable to express as herself, and also that she frequently felt colourless and unnoticed because she so often tried to be good and to do things that would please adults.

Her attitude towards her physical self was reworked in therapy. As we have seen, her general demeanour changed and she walked more confidently, and wore her hair back from her face. Such physical changes are very often direct indications of internal change, an acknowledgement to self and others that new behaviour and new responses are being activated. From the sixth session, when she began to enact her powerful and complex role-plays, Diane often began the session by complaining of physical distress (nausea, headaches), which suggested an intimate link for her between psychic pain and physical pain (a link, incidentally, which points to the aetiology of some psychosomatic complaints as due to unresolved childhood traumas). Not only did her physical abuse give rise to emotional pain but intense negative emotions also seemed to engender real physical distress in her. In the eleventh session, when Diane as the mother slashed red marks down her daughter's entire cheek, Diane's enactment of abuse seemed to show a distortion of her sense of physical identity. The earlier sessions in which Diane made up her face as a witch and as a woman with heavy make-up, who is then punished by her mother for wearing make-up can with hindsight be viewed as being related to Diane's disturbed emotions about her injuries. Her sense of physical impairment seemed closely bound up in her personal, feminine identity.

No facial scarring was in fact visible on Diane; she seemed to have been using facial disfigurement to symbolise her emotional distress to her physical injury. However, in most cases of abuse over a period of time, the extent of this abuse can be hidden and, as Terr (1988) demonstrates and as we discuss further in the chapter on Ben, children do seem to retain long-lasting accurate behavioural memories of bodily injuries and abuses. (Most adults can think of times when they have 'gone cold' with apprehension before consciously knowing what the memory is that is frightening to them.) Her enactment, then, may be of a real experience. Yet perhaps most importantly Diane chose to work through her previous abusive experiences on a physical, motor level, as well as on an emotional and to a lesser extent, cognitive level. A strength of play therapy is that it can be utilised by the child on this physical level, which is a vital one, since early abusive experiences in particular often do not have a cognitive level as their primary one (see also Chapter 6).

A third theme which we identified in Diane's play therapy, is that of her relationship with her brother. As the research cited above indicates, children in abusive settings often develop pseudo-adult behaviours both to placate their caregivers and to pre-empt further abusive behaviours. Such behaviours are often undertaken at the expense of their own needs to be cared for and to be dependent.

Diane's relationship with her younger brother clearly revealed this pattern, showing in her play her ambivalent feelings towards him. She showed how she felt both responsible for protecting him from being injured, and yet rivalrous, because she had to compete with him for the limited adult attention available. In the first of these role-plays, she enacted a physically abusive sequence in which, taking the role of her younger brother, but probably depicting elements of her younger self as well, she was attacked, then limped off to bed and lay very still, refusing all adult help. Her actions conveyed a highly personalised and realistic re-experiencing of physical injury to a defenceless child. This traumatic role-play seemed to depict the way in which Diane felt responsible for caring for her brother in a physically violent household where the adults were dangerous to them. Her task was made even more difficult because her younger brother appeared to her to be demanding and wilful, as well as unaware of his potential danger.

In the later role-plays, she depicted vividly her protective role towards her brother as well as her impatience towards him. She first looked after him, then plotted to get rid of him, and then, faced with the brother's anger, took a doll representing him and tried to disfigure it. It seemed evident that she found it difficult to express her hostility overtly towards people she loved and first resorted to subterfuge and then became enraged and violent when her brother became angry with her. In becoming so angry herself, she seemed to reflect the same abusive pattern of behaviour that her mother had exhibited towards her. This exemplifies the repetitive cycles of abuse between family generations noted in the literature, which we have mentioned above. It should be noted here, however, that the consequences of abuse are *mediated* rather than direct. Kagan (1971), for example, makes a distinction between heterotypical and homotypical continuity of behaviours, suggesting that the child may show the same behaviour as he or she has experienced, but that this may or may not serve the same emotional purposes. The link between the actual experience of abuse and subsequent behaviour is thus a complex one and one needs to be careful about assuming a direct replication of events.

Diane was only able to address her relationship with her mother, which was the most intimate and painful of her difficulties, after her self-confidence and commitment to therapy had increased, although in retrospect earlier actions can be interpreted as circling round this issue. Her role-play in becoming the witch and her mother 'the victim' proved to be a symbolic re-creation of Diane's personal responses, or schemas, for her mother. Through these role-plays, Diane's relatively permanent personal affective, cognitive and motor schemas were re-integrated in a more healthy manner into her current functioning.

In our next chapter, we write about Anna, whose background experiences and personality differed dramatically from Diane's. Anna did, however, like Diane, make use of her play therapy sessions to create a personal, symbolic space within which to work on issues which were of great emotional importance to her.

Chapter 4

Anna

A Silent Communication

I heard the owls, the soft callers, coming down from the hemlocks.
Theodore Roethke, 'I Cry, Love! Love!'

ANNA'S BACKGROUND

Anna was referred to me by her mother, Judith, at the suggestion of Judith's therapist. In our telephone conversation she spoke with concern about the deep unhappiness Anna had been experiencing over the last six months. She was troubled by nightmares and restless sleep, had long bouts of weeping over trivial events, and clung to Judith constantly when they were together. Even though Anna was now seven years old, she seemed to Judith more dependent and demanding than she had ever been before. Judith then explained that she believed Anna's problems were due to the very difficult time their family as a whole was experiencing as a result of divorce proceedings between herself and her estranged husband, Tom. I offered to meet her during the following week to discuss this further and then to decide with her whether I would be able to help Anna.

When we met, Judith immediately became extremely distressed when she began to talk about Anna's unhappiness. She described a typical night with Anna, which usually involved at least one nightmare and a restless sleep pattern; she needed to be settled by her mother each time, after calling out to her up to three or four times during the night. I felt that Judith seemed to have a sensible and well-considered approach to her daughter's sleeping difficulties.

She also appeared to have the kind of stamina and sense of purpose which would help her to keep up the exhausting routine of settling Anna back to sleep night after night. Indeed, she seemed to be able to respond sensitively and appropriately to all Anna's very demanding behaviours. Judith seemed realistically concerned, however, that despite her appropriate responses, Anna had not been able to overcome her troubled behaviour. Judith also admitted to being exhausted by her nightly efforts, and was worried that her own life was restricted, too, by her lack of energy.

We also talked about Anna's earlier childhood. The change in Judith's manner and voice was striking. She now began to relax and smile as she talked about how delightful and easy Anna had been to care for as a baby, how she had been so quick to learn and sweet-natured as a little girl and how thoughtful of others she had always been. While Tom had tended to ignore Daniel, their thirteen year old son, he had had much more time for Anna – he seemed to see Anna as more like himself.

Judith stressed that she wanted her children to keep their relationship with their father and, if possible, to have it improve after their divorce. Her own relationship with Tom, however, had become increasingly frightening for her. He had always seemed at times emotionally cruel to her during their marriage but, since she had left him, he had taken to turning up unexpectedly at her new, smaller house in the neighbourhood to which she had moved with the children, becoming at first verbally and then physically aggressive towards her. As well as pushing her around, repeatedly punching and injuring her, he would usually end his stay by deliberately breaking something of hers as he stormed out of the house. Anna and Daniel had seen all this several times, since Tom seemed to disregard the effect his violence might have on them. Anna especially had seemed very frightened; Daniel a bit less so, perhaps because he was older. Tom was now prevented by a court order from coming to the house and his regular visits to the children had been stopped as well for a while, until things calmed down.

Judith said that she used to talk to the children about their father and had often tried to reassure them that he loved them and was very angry with her, but not with them. Judith added that neither of the children ever talked about him to her any more, so she had been trying not to do so either, since she thought that talking about him might cause them needless worry.

Wondering to myself whether it was also the case that Judith was unable to talk to the children about Tom because of her own fear of him and guilt at leaving him, I observed that maybe they were all three so afraid of Tom's unpredictability and aggression towards her, that none of them found it easy to think or talk about him. Judith listened to me, but did not comment. I also emphasised that it was above all important for Anna and Daniel to know both they and their mother were safe from unexpected attacks from their father, since she was the children's most important person for security now. Judith nodded, adding that her older sister and her brother-in-law had come to live nearby, since her difficulties with Tom had begun. They came to the house frequently, which helped them all feel more secure. However, Tom did still show up at the school gates regularly when she was picking Anna up from school and this was still quite frightening. Judith said she handled this by staying with her friends and ignoring Tom's presence.

Judith was relieved that Daniel, at least, seemed to be coping with all the turmoil and did not have any severe problems. He spent time with his uncle and even more time with his friends; he seemed able to 'get on with his life'.

At this point in our meeting, I had enough information to tell Judith that I was interested in trying to help Anna and moved on to discuss my method of working with children. I also discussed the possible effects on Anna of attending play therapy sessions, stressing Anna's need to feel safe and supported during her sessions. I added that I was hopeful that with the psychological help and family support Judith was now receiving, she would be more able to meet Anna's relating to her father. She already seemed very able to meet many of Anna's other emotional needs.

I said that I would also need to meet Tom myself and talk to him about my method of therapy, and about his past relationship and current feelings towards Anna, to which Judith somewhat reluctantly agreed. I underlined the fact that I would not discuss with him any confidential information that she had shared with me. Our conversation would remain centred on Anna herself, and her father's perceptions and feelings towards her as well as issues which he himself raised. Equally, my discussion with him would remain confidential.

At the end of our meeting we arranged to have another meeting in a month's time to discuss Anna's overall progress; by then Anna would have had time to begin her play therapy sessions. Last, we agreed an initial contract for twenty sessions and Judith signed consent forms for my meetings with other professionals and for audiorecording Anna's sessions (provided the recording did not adversely affect Anna herself).

My subsequent meetings with other professionals and with Anna's father were useful in providing additional dimensions to the knowledge I had received from Judith. The doctor reported that Anna's health was good and her physical health could not account for her symptoms. Her progress academically at school was above average and, although Anna was very shy in her interactions with all of the staff, she seemed able to play well with other children and had no noticeable difficulty making friends. The school was also aware of Anna's unhappiness, having become concerned that, in the classroom, Anna could suddenly withdraw into herself, quietly weeping and becoming for a time inconsolable. They were relieved that I would be seeing Anna.

In my meeting with Tom, I found that his primary emotion in discussing Anna with me was anger with Judith for keeping him apart from his children and ruining his family life. He mentioned the court order barring him temporarily from seeing the children because of his aggression, which he considered to be a great injustice. Judith, he said bitterly, always had managed to get people to feel sorry for her when she put on her 'helpless little girl' act. I acknowledged his deep feelings of hurt and guided the conversation back to Anna's early life and how he felt about her then. Tom described Anna as being much more 'his' than her brother was. She had his personality and she was clever, too. From an early age Anna liked to be near him whenever she could. He'd spent a great deal of time with her, and knew that Anna was always happy in his company and wanted to be with him. She still would be if her mother had not ruined everything.

I talked with him about how angry he still seemed to be with Judith and that I understood that the court had stopped him from seeing his family because he had hurt her in front of their children. Tom denied that his actions had any particular effect on Anna. She had still come close to him and treated him 'just the same'. I replied that several people had told me that in recent months Anna had seemed to be very unhappy. Tom again blamed Judith for Anna's unhappiness, saying all he wanted was to be with his children. They were rightfully his and he intended to fight to get them. I acknowledged the pain he was experiencing, and tentatively wondered if some counselling would be helpful for him, given all that had happened. I realised that he might feel I was 'siding' with Judith because of having been first approached by her, but my main concern was to try and help Anna, who for whatever reason (which might include her pain at being separated from him, or her fear from witnessing his aggression towards her mother) was clearly unhappy. In the long term if he could accept what had happened between himself and Judith, both he and his children would be able to live more peacefully and hopefully begin to build up their relationship with one another again. Tom agreed, somewhat hesitantly, that his children and their happiness were very important to him, and that he would think about what I'd said and perhaps consider getting help for himself.

ANNA'S PLAY THERAPY SESSIONS

After listening to the impressions of Anna from so many concerned adults, I was looking forward to meeting Anna herself to learn from her through play therapy how her life felt from the inside. I called at her home to introduce myself one day early in the week she was scheduled to see me. Anna was silent, looking down at a book on her lap while sitting very close to her mother on the sofa. I began talking to her, saying I had met her mother and she had talked to me about how unhappy Anna seemed to be. She wanted Anna to come to see me in my playroom so that I could try to help her with what worried her.

Anna appeared very uncomfortable as I spoke, so I said that Anna could be feeling that it was difficult to listen to me. Maybe I could tell her mummy about the things Anna might like to know before we started. Addressing myself to Judith, I remarked that Anna might be interested in finding out that I had talked to other people about her coming to see me, too. Her mummy had said that it would be all right for me to talk to Anna's doctor, her daddy and her school. I hoped that it would be all right with Anna to come during schooltime, because it was fine with her mummy and her teacher. I also mentioned the lessons Anna would be missing and said that they had thought those would be the best ones to miss. But Anna could tell her mummy or me if she was unhappy about that. I said that I would leave now; since Judith and I had talked about it already, Anna might want to find out more from her, instead of me, before she came.

I saw Anna arriving outside the building through the family centre window. They had arrived early, with Anna holding her mother's hand tightly; she walked hesitantly and looked apprehensive. Her manner was understandable, yet looked somehow incongruous to me as well, because Anna and her mother both looked very attractive together. They both had short, well-cut, glossy black hair and were dressed in fashionable clothes; their physical appearance conveyed a sense of confidence in themselves and a comfortable lifestyle. I had already prepared the playroom for Anna, and decided that I would write up full notes immediately after her sessions and not use the audiotape in the room, because of her extreme apprehension and silence.

Anna was at the table quietly drawing when I entered the waiting room. Her mother took her to the playroom door, looked inside the room with us and then left, reassuring her that she would be nearby in the waiting room. Anna kept her head down after her mother had left and moved over to the table which had drawing materials, paints and playdough, including cutters and rolling pin, on it. She smiled nervously and looked out of the window rather than at me as I commented that she seemed to have seen something she might like to do. I added that I would sit on the chair near the door and Anna could do anything she wanted.

After hesitantly pulling out a chair, Anna sat down and immediately became engrossed in drawing a picture. She drew a very conventional picture for a girl her age, with blue sky, yellow sun radiating out from the corner of the paper and a red house with yellow windows and door set in the middle of the page. I remained silent; then, as Anna drew a black-haired girl with a smiling face, I commented briefly that the girl was smiling and seemed to like being outside the house. As she elaborately decorated and coloured in the girl's dress, I remarked that the girl was wearing a very nice dress and that Anna wanted her to look nice. Flowers, grass and trees appeared on the other side of the house, but then she drew a black line directly over the house. 'Something black is right on top of the cheerful house and garden', I commented, trying to have a tone of slight apprehension in my voice. Anna hurriedly responded by changing the black line into a multi-coloured rainbow. 'You've made it happy again; you don't want the black over the house', I said quietly. Anna finished her drawing, making a flock of birds and small clouds dot across the sky in a neat row under the original blue line of sky.

Anna looked down at her drawing for a minute or two. 'Maybe you're wondering if you're finished', I remarked. She slowly got up from her chair and brought the drawing over to me, smiling down at the floor in front of her as she handed it to me. I smiled also and commented that she wanted me to see it close up. I looked at it and said to her that she wanted me to see a happy picture with a girl outside the house. Anna had remained silent; now she responded very quietly, 'That's a rainbow'. I replied that I thought it was going to be something black and heavy over the house, but Anna hadn't wanted to leave it that way; she wanted it to be a happy picture with a rainbow. She listened to me as we both looked down at the drawing. (She had avoided meeting my eyes and I consciously tried to respect her way of distancing herself from me.) There was a long pause, with Anna remaining standing in front of me, very still and contained. I commented that maybe she didn't know what to do now. Anna turned away from me, and started to pull up her knee-length socks several times, while beginning to lift her head, looking past the table towards the toys nearby. I said that she didn't seem to be sure what to do next, that she knew that she had wanted to draw, but now she was having a good look at the other toys. She sighed, and a long silence descended, with Anna seeming to be rooted to the spot.

V: You're finding it hard to talk or do anything except stand very still.
A: [Silence and no visible movement]
V: Maybe you've had enough for this time.
A: [Nods]
V: You seem to think you've had enough.
A: I don't want to do anything.
V: You can stay and do nothing – we have a lot of your time left – or go back.
A: Go back.

For her next session, Anna brought along a very small baby doll that fitted in the palm of her hand. She left her mother in the waiting room and came with me by herself. Like her first time, Anna silently chose her activity, this time the sand tray. She began by standing with her back to me as I remained on my chair near the door, then moved after about ten minutes to face me directly, but with her head down, not visibly acknowledging my presence. As she began to dig in the sand, I briefly remarked that she had found something she wanted to do. She silently held her own baby doll in one hand, along with a plastic milkbottle, and used her free hand to fill the bottle's very small opening and neck with wet sand. While I watched her persisting doggedly with this activity, I thought how her actions looked largely futile because only a few grains of sand were going in, with most of it plopping out of the top and landing on the outside of the bottle and in the sand tray. The baby doll in her hand also made the bottle difficult for her to hold. I commented that Anna wanted to fill the bottle, but it was very difficult to do, then added later on that she didn't want to give up, even though it wasn't working out very well for her.

Anna finally put the bottle down, and I said that she had given up now and she must feel tired from trying to make it work for so long. (Since there was no sign of frustration in her manner, I did not reflect this feeling, although I did note to myself that this is the emotion I would have expected a child to show under these circumstances.) Anna began to fill a wide-mouthed bucket with sand, which I commented was very easy for her to do. She patted the sand down in the bucket and levelled it off, making a detailed pattern on top with a rake and spoon handle. As she brought the bucket to show me, I said that she seemed pleased with it and wanted to show me the nice easy things she could do. Anna returned the bucket to the sand, brushed her hands off, still clutching the baby doll, and asked to return to her mother. I responded that we still had a long time, until the big hand of the clock on the wall reached the six, another half-hour, but maybe she didn't want to be with me in the playroom for that long, that she wanted to be with her mummy. Anna nodded, keeping her head down, and we returned to Judith.

At the beginning of her third session, Judith and Anna knocked on the playroom door and came in, having arrived a few minutes late due to a traffic jam on the way into town. I was kneeling down tidying an open shelf filled with different types of drawing paper and Anna joined me silently as her mother left. She immediately began helping me organise all the paper, busy, but uncommunicative. I turned to her after a time and quietly said that we could do it together and that Anna seemed to enjoy sorting things out. Anna made very efficient use of the space on the shelf near her and was a genuine help. For example, she discarded folded or cut pieces of paper appropriately in the waste paper basket, all done without comment or asking my permission first. I commented that she felt she was good at tidying and knew that she could be helpful to me. Anna then went on to find doll's clothes and dressed some of the dolls in a quick and proficient way. When I suggested that she seemed to know how to dress dolls very well too and enjoyed it, Anna talked to me for the first time, replying that she had lots of her own at home. I commented, 'And you take care of them, like you're doing now. Maybe you pretend that you're being a good mummy to them', I added. Anna nodded, continuing to work silently, finished, looked around the room thoroughly, and then nodded. 'You seem pleased with the way things look now', I remarked, and as Anna walked purposely over to the table, sat down and began to draw, I said that she could get on with other things now that the room felt tidy to her.

Anna drew another picture similar to her first one, quietly engrossed in her work, but substituted a bird for the earlier rainbow over her house. This time everything was smiling, including the girl, the sun and the bird. I was shown the drawing, and Anna again stood silently in front of me, appearing to be waiting for my comments. I told her that this picture was a very happy one all the time for everything in her picture. I added 'That's the way you like it, all happy'. Anna nodded and glanced around the room. She then went to the doll's house and silently arranged the furniture, using both sides of the doll's house to make one large house. The furniture was gradually arranged to make functional and attractive rooms – bedrooms, bathrooms, sitting room, kitchen and dining room – much like her own house's layout. Anna spent at least fifteen minutes setting up the doll's house, then quickly put several adults downstairs looking at a television and a couple of children in another room in front of a second television. She then very deliberately closed up the two sides of the doll's house and I commented that she seemed to have sorted it out the way she wanted it. Standing up, Anna looked around the room carefully, this time including me in her glance. I remarked that she was thinking what to do and that her time was almost over, that she had five minutes left today. Anna picked up a doll, held it a moment, and then told me softly she wanted to go back.

The first part of our next session did not seem to carry Anna forward; instead, she seemed to have moved backwards and to be more dependent on her mother. Anna was reluctant to come with me when I went to the waiting room and passively resisted her mother's verbal efforts to persuade her to come with me. I talked about Anna feeling that she needed her mummy very much today and maybe she was trying to tell us she couldn't come on her own. Judith then held her hand and brought her to the playroom. After Judith said goodbye to her at the door, she entered the playroom, but seemed more withdrawn into herself, sucking at the tip of her shirt collar as she drew another 'sunny' picture. I commented that Anna didn't seem to feel very happy to be here herself today, but she still wanted to draw a happy time for herself in the picture. She did not acknowledge my remark and when she finished drawing, instead of bringing her picture to me as before, she sat silently looking down. I remarked that she didn't feel like moving by herself today. She was sitting there, but she didn't seem to like it. (Anna had begun to make small movements in her chair which appeared to be ones of discomfort and restlessness.) 'Maybe', I said, 'you can't think what you want today'. (Anna nodded almost imperceptibly.) 'Maybe it would be easier today if I thought of things to do, then you could choose.' Anna nodded again, keeping her back to me, but this time her nod was slightly more noticeable. I said that other times she chose the sand and doll's house – Anna did not glance at them or move, remaining impassive – but maybe today she wanted something different. I pointed out the musical instruments and the zoo animals on their own board that she might look at. Instead she silently moved over to the doll's house and again spent the rest of the hour until the time was up arranging all the furniture into rooms in a large house, but this time having large pauses looking into space between many of her movements. Near the end of her hour she placed a woman with a man watching television downstairs, while the two children were placed upstairs in bedrooms. I spoke little myself during this play, confining myself to a few quiet comments on Anna needing to think a lot about what she was doing and the children being on their own upstairs while the big people were together downstairs. Anna closed the house in a thoughtful manner and silently returned to her mother at the end of the hour.

During the following week Judith and I met as planned to discuss Anna's progress. Judith felt hopeful that Anna could be helped, noticing that, although Anna had been very clingy at times, she had decided to start dance classes again and wanted to go along to them with her friend and the friend's mother. Anna had also taken to finding her new baby doll when she woke up in the night and sometimes seemed to settle herself back to sleep. She did, though, still have a recurring nightmare several times a week. Judith said that this nightmare had changed and no longer was of monsters coming to take her away. She was now dreaming that a man was running into her bedroom and trying to pull her out of bed. Judith said she didn't question Anna on who the man was, just saying no one would take her away. However, Judith thought it could be Tom that Anna was dreaming about. I replied that I thought she was making the right responses. I also told Judith that Anna seemed to be able to make use of the time we had together, but that it was apparent that it was difficult for her to come. I was pleased that Judith was able to stay during the hour in order to enable Anna to keep her own pace and not have to stay longer than she could manage. I added that Judith's presence still seemed very important for Anna's sense of security.

Anna's next session, her fifth, was a very industrious one for her. She organised materials, including paper, paints, playdough and felt tips, as I remarked that she wanted to do everything for herself today. Remaining silent and with her back to me at the table, Anna experimented with different materials on her paper. Instead of a happy outdoor scene, Anna used playdough and playdough cutters to cut out shapes, then paint and felt tips to join together the cutouts and to decorate them with designs and faces. She seemed to have no emotion other than industriousness today, which I acknowledged by my remarks about Anna being very busy and being interested in how she could use the different things in her picture. At the end of the hour, after I had already told Anna that we would have to finish soon, she stopped, gave me a brief direct look, and told me that she was ready to go.

Anna again held back from coming with me for our sixth session. Judith was surprised at her reaction and said that Anna had been telling her how she wanted to talk with me about her daddy. I repeated to Anna that she could do and say what she wanted, like she always did in the playroom; she could come along and see what she felt like doing. Anna silently came with me and immediately sat down at the table to draw. She drew another happy picture of sky, sun and house, garden with flowers blooming and a black-haired girl outside. This time, however, the girl's mouth was black; it seemed distorted, and too large for the face. I commented that her picture was a happy one, but there seemed to be something wrong with the girl's mouth. Anna put that drawing aside on the table and got another piece of paper from the shelf. She used paint thickly to make a very black house. I commented that Anna had made a big house and it was very dark and gloomy. She then painted the sun in the corner and I said that she didn't want everything to be black, that it was still sunny outside. Anna got up and handed me the painting when she finished. I commented on how dark and light were together now in her painting and began to hand it back to her as I usually did. But Anna fixed her gaze on my hand and shook her head slightly, keeping her hands by her sides. 'You want me to keep this one, then', I replied, and Anna nodded, then told me quietly she was going back to her mummy. I said that it was early, but she'd had enough today.

Our next session was even more difficult for Anna to begin. She clung to her mother very tightly when her mother led her to the playroom door, and would not let go of her arm. Anna's desperation was very evident and I said that she wanted her mummy very much today and seemed to feel frightened without her. Judith registered my comment and accompanied us inside the playroom. She sat down in my chair and Anna crawled into her lap and sucked at the corner of her shirt; for a while Judith held her close. I talked about Anna needing her mummy especially close to her today, letting Anna feel enclosed in and comforted by her mother's embrace. I also said how nice and warm and peaceful it felt when her mummy held her close like that. In a short time Anna began to get a bit restless in Judith's arms, which was a signal for Judith to say that it was time for her to get a drink. Protesting a bit, Anna was put down and Judith left, reassuring Anna that she would be in the waiting room when she had finished.

Anna spent some time standing where she was put down and looking around the room. After playing silently with the tea set, she crossed the room to the doll's house and once again played with the doll figures and furniture until the end of the hour. This time, instead of one large house, she divided each side into two smaller ones. Using all the child and adult figures available, she found places for all the children in the bedrooms and all the adults in downstairs rooms of both houses. A girl then came down the stairs and began to speak in a clear voice, asking: 'Mummy, please can I stay downstairs and watch TV with everybody?' The adult figure silently refused (Anna shook her head, rather than speaking for the adult) and brought the girl back upstairs, then went downstairs and joined the other adults. The girl turned over and went to sleep. During all these silent actions by Anna, I became the narrator, commenting first that the girl didn't want to be by herself in the bedroom and later that the girl could go to sleep by herself, and the mummy wanted to go and be with the other big people. Internally, I was fascinated by this transition in Anna's play, noting that the girl doll had been released from her silence by Anna, allowing me in turn to become a more active narrator.

In our eighth session, Anna's manner was very different. She seemed determined to begin it quickly. After marching ahead of me and entering the playroom first, Anna smiled confidently as she looked around the room. I commented that she felt very sure about everything today. She smiled at me briefly and sank down on the floor next to the musical instruments. As she removed the drums, cymbals and tambourine from their basket, she tentatively tried the drumsticks on each instrument in turn. Wondering what they sound like, I murmured, as Anna made very soft sounds. I also reassured her that children were allowed to make a noise in the playroom if they wanted to, but that maybe Anna wanted just quiet sounds.

Anna tidied the instruments away after a short time, this whole play sequence being done confidently but without speaking, and turned to play with the zoo nearby. She began to concentrate, sorting the animals silently into groupings and placing each group into separate areas and buildings on the zoo's board. The monkeys were given preferential treatment: they had their own building and rocks, a pool, and a fence separating their large space from the rest of the zoo animals. I remarked to her on their nice place in the zoo. She then placed all the monkeys outside in their enclosed area and had a male lion climb up on the fence. The monkeys were all put into the building quickly, but two small monkeys remained on the rocks outside. A big monkey came out, which she made bob its head excitedly at the little ones, and brought them inside. I commented that the big one seemed cross with the little ones for being outside; it seemed dangerous for all the monkeys because a big lion was nearby. Anna then had the lion try to climb the fence in several places, while the big monkey frantically ran around the enclosed area, following the lion's movements. I said in a worried tone that the big monkey was trying to keep everyone safe, but had to be watching all the time. The lion did succeed in entering after a time and knocked down the big monkey, then returned to its own section of the zoo board. 'The big monkey's hurt', I said in a concerned way, 'but all the other monkeys are safe for now.'

Anna repeated this scene two more times, with the smaller monkeys watching the big monkey, who tried to protect them and each time got hurt. I commented on how it was happening so much, that the little ones must be very frightened every time they see the big one hurt. This sequence was acted out a fourth time, but this time the monkeys had recruited two large elephants to come into their enclosure and remain with the large monkey, while the lion again tried to find a place to climb the fence. I said in a relieved voice that the monkey had found some big ones to help her, as Anna made the elephants and monkey bar the lion's path after the lion had managed to scale the fence. The animals then joined together to drive the lion far away, first to the other end of the zoo and then completely off the zoo board. The elephants followed the lion, knocking it down and stamping on it, while the monkey returned to the little ones. I conveyed an enormous sense of relief in my voice as the action finished, saying with feeling that the little ones had the big one back, and this time, not hurt! It was the lion that got hurt for being bad to the monkey and was sent away by the big elephants. Anna looked up at me as I finished talking, smiling with pleasure. I returned her smile: 'You feel better now', I said warmly, and Anna nodded, her smile widening for me and her eyes shining.

She glanced at the clock and saw that her hour was almost over. Leaving the rest of the zoo as she had arranged it, she took out one of the small monkeys and placed it in my hand, again smiling deeply into my eyes. Then she opened the door and skipped ahead of me to her mother in the waiting room. Anna surprised me further by loudly calling 'goodbye' to me as I left the waiting room. I realised, as I walked back to the playroom and thought about our intensive time, that my inner reaction to her 'goodbye' was so strong, not merely because she had never before spoken in a loud voice, but even more because this was the first word Anna had spoken to me during our entire hour together.

My next meeting with Judith was scheduled to follow this session with Anna. Before our meeting I talked with Judith's therapist, who felt optimistic about the progress she was making in working through her unrealistic guilt and her sense of sole responsibility for her divorce. Judith also was beginning to develop her own life apart from Tom and from her family, which gave her increased confidence, he felt, in coping with both Tom's behaviour and with the children on her own.

Judith was eager to talk with me when she came about all that had happened in the last month. She began by saying that her own life was improving and that seemed to be helping Anna. It certainly made a difference that Anna was beginning to sleep much better, with only an occasional nightmare. Having a good night's sleep herself gave her much more energy. She still had a lot of problems with Tom, but he seemed to be fighting her more indirectly – their joint property and other financial issues had become grounds for protracted legal arguments. However, Judith added, she'd decided to let her solicitor worry about all these headaches for now. Judith then concentrated on Anna, wondering if I felt it was all right that Anna was starting to talk to her, just in the last week or so, about her daddy. Weren't those the kinds of things that were important for Anna to talk to me about instead? I assured her that I thought this was a very positive step and that I certainly didn't think Anna should talk exclusively to me about her feelings. On the contrary, it was important, since Anna felt very close to her mother, that she could choose to talk to her. Judith said that they seemed able to talk a bit about better times they all had had in the past. I pointed out that Anna might be feeling that it wouldn't cause her mother too much pain now if they talked together about her father. Judith said that Anna certainly *had* begun to talk about painful times. She had said that she remembered Tom hitting Judith and how frightened she felt. Judith confessed that she hadn't known how to respond and so she hadn't said anything. I suggested she might want to talk about her own feelings that Anna might be arousing in her with her therapist and added that the question of Anna's future contact with her father would clearly need to be thought through also. She was more able to express her anger with him now, but would need at some point to be able to express the undoubtedly positive feelings she had had about him, too, and hopefully to be helped to re-establish a relationship with him sometime. What was important for Anna first of all, I felt, was that her mother had been able to listen to and accept her strong feelings, and that Anna was probably feeling safer, and more confident in Judith's power to protect her. Judith nodded without speaking. After a pause, she talked proudly about Anna's new gregariousness and confidence with adults, which was even noticed by her teacher at school.

I then said that Anna seemed to be making such good progress that perhaps five or ten more sessions with me would be enough for her. I also added that I raised this possibility because of thinking that Anna's parents might take some time to be able to re-establish a new kind of viable partnership concerning the children, well beyond the amount of time it would be useful for Anna to work individually with me. I would recommend Judith and Tom making use of the family conciliation service in town. Judith became immediately concerned, saying she felt unready to be Anna's only emotional support, and she didn't know if Tom could change. I offered to meet monthly with Judith after my work with Anna ended in order to talk over Judith's concerns about Anna and to check that Anna seemed to be maintaining her emotional progress. Judith agreed with some relief. I also stressed, however, that I did not want to rush into ending if Anna indicated to me or to Judith that she needed more sessions. We decided to leave the issue of ending open for now and judge from Anna's reactions in the next few weeks what the appropriate decision would be. We ended our meeting in a relaxed way, with Judith chatting easily and finding me a very receptive audience for her details about Anna's daily life.

Before Anna's ninth session I was even more intrigued than usual by what would emerge during our next session, given the intensity of our previous time together. Anna came into the playroom for our session readily, and although not talkative, seemed relaxed and easy in my presence. She told me she was going to do a special picture, and spent her entire time working on a large collage of flowers and trees in a garden. The picture was made from sticky paper and glued crepe paper of different colours and joined together using felt-tip pens. I commented that Anna liked thinking about everything outside in the garden and how she enjoyed working on a picture that was very big with lots of different kinds of lovely things in it. After looking at the clock and noticing that she had ten minutes left, Anna quickly finished her picture and began to wash her hands and tidy up.

As she worked industriously, I briefly talked to her about how we'd had nine times in the playroom now and after ten times with children, I think about whether more times are a good idea or not. Anna seemed a lot happier and not so worried now. Anna nodded. She could come more times if she needed to, I reassured her; I would be in the playroom for her. Maybe we could both think about it and decide together next week. Anna listened to me as she tidied up, glancing at me from time to time as I spoke, but not responding. Having finished her work, she picked up her picture and held it carefully in front of herself, with both hands outstretched to accommodate such a large picture. She allowed me to go in front of her, opening the doors for her as she carried her picture proudly back to her mother. As I left Anna was talking with animation to Judith, who was listening with appreciation, about how she had managed to construct her elaborate picture.

For our tenth session, Anna walked into the playroom and, without hesitation, went directly over to the sand tray. She added some water from the sink, making the sand damp and malleable. Making hills and valleys, Anna used a spade to dig out roads on the hillsides and built up mounds of sand for bridges spanning the valleys. Then putting a man figure into one of the plastic cars from the tray nearby, she drove it up and down the roads she'd engineered, with the car getting stuck and the road needing to be constantly rebuilt as she moved the car and driver along. I commented briefly that the road was out in the hills, maybe in the countryside, as she built it, and then commented on how difficult it was for her to have the man and his car move along the road. Anna had to work hard for a very long time to let them go along it.

Anna started to drive the man in the car very fast over the hills, made the car crash in a valley and get buried in the sand. I remarked that the man had disappeared; Anna then quickly started digging holes in the hills which were furthest away from the crashed car. I said that she was looking, but she wouldn't find the car there. Anna then moved over to dig up the driver and car, looked very crossly at it and threw it back in its hole in the sand. 'You look very cross; you don't want to see him. You're *cross* with him', I commented in a quiet but angry tone of voice. Anna then dug up the man and car, putting them back in the tray nearby. 'You're finished with that', I said with the same emphasis in my voice that Anna had used in her placement of the toys in the tray. Anna looked across at me and nodded in a definite manner. 'I want to go back to my mummy now', she said, after looking at the clock and seeing that her hour was only half-finished. I mentioned our thinking today about having more times together and what we both want. Anna remained silent and I added that I'd like to see her more times, because she still seemed to need to play in here with me, like today. Anna shook her head slightly. I asked. 'Maybe you've had enough times in here with me?' Anna nodded seriously at me. 'I'll see your mummy a few more times to talk with her, Anna, and see you again, maybe after you've had a rest from the playroom for a while?' Anna nodded, smiled at me briefly and we returned to her mother. I repeated my last remarks to Judith, who immediately assured her that was fine for her too. We all said goodbye until later and as I returned to the playroom and began to put some of the toys back on the higher shelves, I felt somewhat wistful and realized that I would have preferred to continue seamlessly the silent, yet intense and satisfying communication we had developed together, especially during our last few sessions; I now had to accept that this pace did not suit Anna, who needed a 'sabbatical' for a while.

Epilogue

I had a further group of five sessions with Anna a few months later. I have not heard now from Anna's mother for eighteen months – a very hopeful sign in this particular case. While I do not know the outcome of Anna's relationship with her father, Judith had intended to attempt to engage with Tom on this issue with help from their local conciliation service.

PRACTICE ISSUES

Working with silence

It is well recognised in the therapeutic literature that a client's pauses and silences are important communications and need to be used effectively by the therapist (e.g. Casement, 1985). Non-verbal and verbal communications, or 'emotive' messages (see Heard and Lake, 1986), which convey participants' feelings, thoughts and wishes to one another, are also essential components of any therapeutic dialogue. However, with some clients, and especially with children, non-verbal communication and emotive messages may become the primary mode of interaction in therapy. Rather than using toys and other symbolic means to clarify verbalisations, the child's actions, the toy objects and symbols are dominant and are used in lieu of speech, as in Anna's therapy sessions.

Clients' ability to communicate deeply on a verbal level to themselves and others about their inner lives may be inhibited for a variety of reasons. They may have readily apparent physical or mental handicaps, which make speech difficult or impossible for them (see Kennedy, 1995, writing about deaf children and Sinason, 1992, on mentally handicapped clients). In addition, their normal developmental immaturity may mean that they have not yet developed the mental resource of inner speech (Vygotsky, 1962) or the verbal skills necessary for more complex communication with others (see chapter 2). In other cases, such as Anna's, reasons for the silence are not as immediately apparent. The therapist had hypothesised at referral that her young age and developmental regression might be offset in part by a higher than normal intelligence, resulting in a greater ability to verbalise her thoughts and feelings than children normally possess at seven years of age. There had been no reports of suspected hearing loss and she appeared able to speak fluently in other contexts. When the therapist met Anna, however, she quickly saw that her hypothesis was untenable; she was presented with an abnormally silent child.

The therapist's hypotheses of Anna's reasons for silence and ideas of ways to work effectively with her within this silence needed to evolve in the sessions through cues from Anna herself. A variety of reasons for Anna's silence emerged: one possibility was that this behaviour was an indication of her unwillingness to attend, yet her engrossed activity within the sessions and her ability to indicate when she had had enough seemed to make this implausible.

In the referral meeting with Judith, the therapist had hypothesised (to herself) that Anna might be unable to talk about her father to her mother because the latter found it difficult to facilitate this. Judith had also said at the referral that some of the injuries inflicted by Tom had been around her mouth. The therapist speculated that Anna might have seen her mother physically unable to talk to her, as well as emotionally unreachable on the topic of her father, because of these injuries. She also hypothesised, drawing on principles of child development, that Anna would be closely identified with her mother, a view that later evidence in the sessions confirmed. This identification with her mother, linked with her mother's actual and emotional difficulty in speaking about these highly charged concerns, might have inhibited Anna from speaking during her sessions. It also became clearer as her sessions continued that she had witnessed, and been very frightened by, the violent events between her parents, perhaps to the point of having been rendered horrified and 'speechless' about them.

Another reason for Anna's initial silence seemed possibly to be bound up with her personality structure – she was a quiet, thoughtful child and did not readily seem to feel at ease with unfamiliar adults. Yet information from other sources indicated that she was articulate and not overly inhibited once a situation became familiar to her. Given that Anna was able to speak well in other circumstances, another possibility the therapist needed to consider was whether at some level she was perhaps hiding thoughts, events and her deeper feelings from both herself and from others (especially adults).

The nature of the relationships which Anna experienced with carers and other professionals was relevant in exploring whether Anna's silence suggested this kind of concealment (or denial). A very general working rubric for evaluating a child's emotional distance from adults is whether the child has an adult she shares time with and discloses feelings to, and whether generally both the child and this adult have positive, and to a much lesser extent, negative feelings towards one another (Healy et al., 1990). Applying this framework to Anna's relationships, she appeared to be very emotionally close to her mother, and not as close to her father. However, she did not seem able to acknowledge or express any negative emotions to her mother, only positive ones, at the beginning of her therapy sessions. By the end of her ten sessions, Anna was able to express negative feelings about her father to her mother, but not any positive ones. Also, she still did not seem able to feel or express any negativity towards her mother, perhaps because she felt so insecure and so dependent on her at this period. Thus, since expressing positive *and* negative feelings towards both her parents, in different ways, was so troubling for her, this could have been a further reason for her silence in a setting where she was addressing emotionally charged concerns.

One final emotional meaning for Anna of silence seemed to be that she was giving the emotive message that her mother was the primary person she needed to fulfil her emotional needs related to her father. She seemed to be hiding verbal messages about her father from the therapist, as a person of lesser emotional importance to her than her mother. The therapist in turn respected Anna's emotional distancing from her through silence and did not attempt to persuade her to talk, or probe with Anna the reasons for her silence. Not only can a child's ability to talk about events lag behind the child's symbolic communications, it is also crucial for therapists to accept and act on the premise that not all emotional roles should be or need to be fulfilled by her.

Certainly, as we stress in chapter 5 (and earlier in Wilson et al., 1992; Wilson, 1993; Ryan et al., 1995), the main attachment role needs to be fulfilled by the child's daily carer. Yet as Heard and Lake (1986) have outlined in their theoretical model of the attachment dynamic, the therapist still was used emotionally by Anna in an important way. It was through the therapist's emotional support that Anna was able to restore her own confidence and become more self-reliant. She was then able to move forward developmentally and participate more fully in a normal attachment relationship with her mother.

No single one of these possible explanations could ever be proved to be 'right', and indeed, for the most part, they provided ways of helping to identify possible themes and concerns for Anna, all of which may have been accurate at one point or another, and of thinking through how best to respond to her. One of the hypotheses helped the therapist, for example, to be alert and responsive to Anna's difficulty in holding both positive and negative feelings together, as when she gave her 'black' picture to the therapist to keep. [Jane Campion's account of the silent heroine in *The Piano*, although somewhat fragmentary, provides a fictional account of silence which is never fully understood. It is interesting in that it describes a girl, Ada, who at approximately the same age as Anna, became mute as a result of shame at a public rebuke from her father, and seems for many years thereafter to have found her piano an adequate way of communicating emotionally with the world, without others or indeed Ada herself ever fully understanding what prompted her continuing silence. (See Wilson and Ridler, 1996, for a further discussion of childhood attachment themes expressed in literature.)]

Respecting a child's emotional defences against memories of events which cause deep anxiety, a principle of play therapy we discussed in chapters 1 and 3, included in Anna's case respecting her need for silence and not urging her to speak. The therapist did not, however, require Anna to remain in the playroom for the entire hour either, since this also seemed to cause her anxiety. Nor did the therapist remain passive, which could well have been interpreted by Anna as a lack of concern and understanding of her difficulties. She actively encouraged Anna to remain there and helped her to find activities to move her forward, rather than allowing her to feel 'stuck', and unable to move both physically and metaphorically.

The therapist's principal role emotionally during the sessions developed into one in which the therapist became Anna's 'inner voice'. We have already referred to children being in the process of developing 'inner speech', in which language becomes not only an external means for a child of regulating his or her actions, and communicating needs to others, but also becomes an internal means of self-communication (Vygotsky, 1962). At seven a child is usually able internally to represent uncomplicated thoughts and actions, but not more complex ones. Anna's feelings and thoughts towards family members and events were, as her sessions illustrate, very complex as well as being emotionally highly laden. Gilligan notes the emotive power and meaning of a person's voice:

> ... by voice I mean something like what people mean when they speak of the core of the self. Voice is natural and also cultural. It is composed of breath and sound, words, rhythm, and language. And voice is a powerful psychological instrument and channel, connecting inner and outer worlds. Speaking and listening are a form of psychic breathing. (1993: xvi)

Two episodes in Anna's therapy seemed particularly significant in this respect. When the therapist put into words first Anna's symbolic representations with the zoo animals and then with the man in the car, Anna listened intently and the therapist became akin to Anna's 'inner voice', articulating her inner self. Anna was immersed in her enactment, yet aware that the therapist was aiding her self-discovery, with the result that she seemed to feel at those moments perfectly understood and valued, with a profound inner sense of self-worth and happiness. These feelings in a client seem to fit the criteria for peak moments of life experiences (Maslow, 1970, Mahrer and Nadler, 1986) and are believed by Rogers

(1976) to be the ingredients necessary for significant personality change.

In using Anna's story to illustrate the ways in which a therapist can help a child in play therapy have meaningful, but mostly silent communication, we have selected the points in Anna's sessions where the therapist felt Anna required verbal responses and appropriate actions from her. Some of the details in our account of her sessions also highlight other issues for practice. First, in working with a child who remains silent, the therapist must be very observant of minute behaviours of the child and see these as essential communications (see also Wilson et al., 1992: chapter 4). Additionally, she needs to link and compare these behaviours to patterns of behaviour exhibited earlier by the child in order to note differences and similarities from session to session, and thus to be alert to the possible significance of any changes. There are a number of instances in Anna's story which illustrate this process. One example is when Anna kept her hands at her sides in session six rather than stretching them out to take her picture back. This unusual absence of movement led the therapist to link Anna's black house with her knowledge that Anna wanted to hold on only to happy emotions, and to deduce from this that Anna might want her to keep it.

As our description of Anna's sessions may convey, a child's silence can initially be an intimidating mode of communication for the therapist. While it is crucial for the therapist to examine carefully whether her responses and attitudes have contributed to this response in a child, it is possible for the therapist to become too self-critical, not realising that some of her own anxiety is being heightened by the anxiety of the child. She can become hesitant and paralysed herself and miss the relevance of silent communication from the child. Especially for beginning therapists, a child's lack of overt response may heighten the natural feelings of inadequacy which arise from inexperience and a growing sense of panic may pervade the therapist's responses to the child. These feelings may be counterproductive for an already anxious child. The therapist's anxious emotive message may easily convey itself to the child, resulting in the child panicking further and even at times resulting in a breakdown in therapy.

If the therapist is able to accept silence not as a failure to communicate, but as one way of communicating, then it ceases to be disabling, and the child, too, experiences acceptance and reassurance and is freed to explore other means of expression, as Anna did with increasing intensity. We discuss in chapter 1 the importance of close supervision, particularly for beginning therapists. When working with a silent child, this can be vital for all therapists, providing them with additional support and a means of working through the child's and their own potentially ambiguous emotive messages and defences.

Having experience with non-verbal children to draw on can increase therapists' confidence in working with silent children. Parents of infants, for example, must respond on a daily basis to non-verbal communications and build up a repertoire of possible responses based on their knowledge of the child's experiences and past needs, which is in some ways similar to the sensitised responses of the play therapist to the silent child's needs (Schaffer, 1989; see also chapter 2, Patrick). Children who are mentally impaired or have hearing difficulties also rely more heavily on non-verbal communication, and working with them teaches the therapist to be highly observant of and adept at using different forms of communication.

In fact, working with Anna was much easier in terms of communication than working with very young or impaired children. Anna could and did speak when she wished to and she always understood what the therapist said to her. Speech, therefore, was used in a very meaningful way, primarily by the therapist, and as the sessions progressed, Anna increasingly trusted the therapist to understand her emotive messages without her having spoken. One of many examples occurred in her fourth session: Anna remained in her chair, restlessly moving around in it, instead of getting up and bringing her picture over to show the therapist, as she had done previously. The therapist asked herself whether Anna wanted to stay in the room, yet was unable to know what to do herself because she was so anxious. For this reason the therapist tentatively suggested activities and toys to her, but deliberately confined herself to the things in the room Anna had already used or been interested in, and without suggesting to her how to use them. The development of Anna's trust in the therapist's understanding of her emotional life gradually developed, and culminated in session eight, in the sequence with the zoo animals, in which her non-verbal actions were clarified and shared intimately between them both. An intensely personal dialogue had been set up, with Anna's 'gift' of the monkey interpreted by the therapist privately as Anna's deliberately symbolic, silent way of thanking the therapist for releasing a part of herself.

The therapist's role, as it would be with other, less silent children, was at times either to reinforce and make more concrete feelings and events Anna was experiencing during the sessions or to link together two or more emotions Anna seemed to have kept emotionally isolated from one another. For example, the therapist talked about the adults being downstairs and the children upstairs when Anna played in the doll's house, confining herself, as she would with a more verbal child, to reflecting first the child's feeling at not wanting to be on her own, and then her feeling, when brought back upstairs, that she could go to sleep now and her mother could go downstairs again. In commenting thus, the therapist asked herself privately whether Anna's fear concerning her mother's beatings by her father could be connected with the prominence Anna gave this play sequence. Judith had already told the therapist that she was beginning to socialise again, perhaps reactivating Anna's fear for her mother's safety when her mother was not near her upstairs at night. The therapist in her comments sometimes does not reach even this level of provisional understanding of the child's play sequences (as we discuss in Patrick's chapter), and the therapist was, as she responded, conscious of other possible levels of meaning to the sequence, for example, that the two houses perhaps represented her father's house and their own, and a wish for them to be adjacent. Although it can at times feel somewhat unnerving not to have inner certainty and precision, the therapist is guided by her aim of making her comments relevant but not restrictive of the child's free exploration of emotional issues. Some minimal verbalisation of the play activity seems essential in helping the child anchor the experience and the emotions involved, but overspecificity may either be inaccurate, or limit or foreclose the child's exploration. It may also provide too direct a challenge to the child's defences, an issue we discuss in the following section.

Non-directive approaches then view verbalisation on the part of the child as one of the many ways in which a child can express thoughts and feelings (e.g. Moustakas, 1959). The value of talking is not seen to lie so much in the contents of the child's words as in the child's freedom to engage in talk itself. Anna's story illustrates another variation: in her therapeutic intervention, the therapist rather than the child herself was the one who through words made the child's feelings more manageable and concrete. This process is identical, we think, to that described in our accounts of play activities with other children in this book, where the therapist tries to articulate in a tentative way what the child is expressing in the sequence. Anna's silence perhaps served to highlight and intensify this function.

Reworking traumatic memories in therapy

Whether or not highly personal material must be verbalised if therapy is to be effective has been frequently debated in the therapuetic literature. Approaches which are more interventionist, including psychoanalytic approaches, often adopt this viewpoint (see Ross, 1959; Chethik, 1989; Gil, 1991). This is particularly so in relation to working therapeutically with traumatised children, where different approaches have been proposed (see, for example, Pynoos and Eth, 1986; Terr, 1990; Gil, 1991; Hendricks et al., 1993). Pynoos and Eth advocate active direction of the child by the therapist immediately after a traumatic event in order to help the child face such an overwhelming experience, rather than allowing the child to build up strong, but ultimately maladaptive, defences against the event. Also, in cases where the child has been repeatedly traumatised or where defences such as post-traumatic enactments or behaviour have already developed, it is argued that the therapist should form a therapeutic relationship with the traumatised child in order to facilitate the clinician's 'gentle probing to assist the child in addressing intolerable emotions' (Gil, 1991: 75).

In non-directive play therapy, however, as Anna's case illustrates, the therapist does not attempt to make the child face his or her terrifying emotions and memories directly. Anna was allowed to maintain her stance of consciously accepting only happy emotions, leaving her defences intact. It was important, though, that the therapist did note and comment on the negative 'black line' when it appeared in her picture and then on other 'black' and frightening feelings. A non-directive therapist, as we have discussed, tries to comment on the feelings that the child is currently experiencing in a non-threatening manner, rather than remaining a passive observer. In play or behaviour re-enactments as well, a non-directive play therapist would comment on, or (as, say, with Diane, chapter 3), physically take part in the re-enactments as directed by the child, thus allowing the child to arrive at his or her own new solutions in the process of assimilating an overwhelming past experience (Chethik, 1989). In this sense the non-directive play therapist takes 'an active role in helping the child both enter and manoeuvre the play, a role of actively commenting, rearranging, or intruding upon the sequence of events the child portrays. Re-experiencing alone is not enough' (Gil, 1991: 75).

Reworking of a traumatic experience in therapy, however, does not need, as we stated above, to include a verbal response on the part of the child, as Anna's play sequences demonstrate. For a young child, in particular, mental awareness may take the form of mental imagery or other external symbolic representations such as paintings or play scenes (see Wilson et al., 1992: chapter 2).

Both the non-directive and the more directive approaches do, however, share the psychodynamic assumption that in order for a child to recover full emotional health:

> ... the trauma must eventually be brought into awareness and put into perspective, or the repressed memories will appear in the form of intrusive thoughts, nightmares, reenactments, or emotional problems. (Gil, 1991: 77)

In Anna's life her strong emotional defence against unhappiness and fear seemed to result in nightmares, restless sleep, clinging to her mother and emotional numbing as well as weepiness. As she began consciously to accept her negative emotions, her behavioural difficulties abated.

Ending therapy

The third practice issue we wish to address in Anna's sessions concerns the ending of therapy: what are the indications that it is time to draw the therapy sessions to an end? We have already discussed this topic in our previous book (pp. 129–134), pointing out that, since there will always be some outstanding problems remaining, the decision is often, or indeed usually, based on a balancing of the gains and risks in doing so:

> with children who have difficult lives, some basic conflicts will seem to go unresolved [at the end of their sessions]. The advantages of the child feeling independent and able to deal with his own problems without therapeutic help, which termination of therapy clearly states to him, must be weighed against how important the child's problems still seem to himself, his carers and his school . . . the therapist must decide when progressive development is again spontaneously under way in a child and seems likely to be sustained. (Wilson et al., 1992: 130)

In Anna's case, it seemed that by the end of the first ten sessions, one of the principal objectives, which had emerged early on in her therapy, namely allowing her to become sufficiently emotionally independent of her mother to resolve her acute anxiety about her mother's and her own safety, had been met. There were indications in Anna's behaviour outside therapy which suggested that she was now much less troubled. Her mother, helped by her own therapy and Anna's better emotional state, also seemed better equipped to respond to any further troubles. We explore these issues below, as well as considering possible contraindications to concluding her therapy.

The therapist had accepted from early on the limited role that Anna had given her in her emotional life. It was clear throughout that Anna wished her mother to help her with important emotional issues, and it did not seem likely or necessary that Anna develop a long-term relationship with the therapist. Anna's close relationship with her mother had many positive features and her mother cared for her sensitively and appropriately. However, at the outset of therapy, Anna and her mother appeared, because of the family problems, to be more involved with one another than was appropriate for Anna's stage of development. A goal of therapy thus became to increase the emotional breadth of their relationship so that it could include Anna's difficult emotions concerning her father, and decrease Anna's anxious dependency on her mother.

When Anna began to make use of help from the therapist, she did so by exploring some of her negative feelings about life within her home, and her anxieties about her mother's and her own safety. In doing so she seemed to become less at the mercy of these hidden feelings, less frightened and thus less dependent emotionally upon her mother. This was evidenced in her being able to sleep through the night, allowing her mother an adult life independent from her, and in her decision to go to a new dance class with a friend. Anna's progress within therapy sessions was not a steady progression towards independence; for example, she regressed to the behaviour of a very young child in sitting on her mother's knee and sucking her collar at the beginning of one of her sessions. Nonetheless, within this same session, she was able to explore the meaning to her of her mother remaining downstairs with other adults in the evening when Anna was in bed. (It is worth noting that children at times express great anxiety before embarking on a particularly intense sequence of activity.) Anna did not as a result of her increasing independence seem to increase her dependence on the therapist but seemed able to sustain this level of emotional independence herself: another indication that she was readying herself to end therapy.

There were other signs of her greater emotional well-being, both within the sessions, where she became increasingly able to display a wide range of emotions appropriately (for example, in the ninth session in her industriousness and pleasure in producing a large painting), and also in school, where she was reported to be much happier, and no longer tearful and withdrawn. There had, of course, always been signs that in some areas of her life, Anna was functioning adequately. Her ability to sustain friendships with children of her own age as well as her ability to maintain superior academic work in spite of her emotional distress were signs of normal development. It seems likely that Anna's higher than average intelligence, while perhaps forcing her to be aware of more details and emotions connected with her family's distress, also was a factor in her resilience. It allowed her to maintain a more than adequate level of performance at school and very probably helped her to make good use of her sessions so quickly.

Finally, another important reason for considering ending sessions with Anna, as we have implied above, is that Anna herself was strongly communicating with the therapist that the sessions had served some of their purpose for her in her current life, with the threatening lion vanquished and the drawing of the large sunny picture. Her negative feelings to the man and car were very strong, however, and seemed to be signalling a new, more direct way of symbolising her feelings for her father. These seemed especially painful for her, when she buried the man and his car, then put them firmly away. The therapist judged that her distress was very deep-seated, yet perhaps not yet amenable to intervention because of her parents' continuing conflict, hence the suggestion of a pause in their sessions before a planned series leading to a final ending. As we have already stated:

> The therapist, while the appropriate one to make the decision about ending, must try to understand the child's viewpoint and as far as possible make the decision a joint one. (Wilson et al.,1992: 130)

The therapist's intention was thus to help Judith distinguish, should further problems arise at a later stage, whether she could help Anna herself, as was to be hoped, or whether more play therapy sessions were necessary.

During the course of their next five sessions the therapist clearly recognised that there were issues that still remained unresolved at the end of Anna's therapy. In particular, although Anna's anger with her father had surfaced, her positive feelings about him and her feelings of loss, had not found expression. In some areas of her emotional life, she had been able, symbolically, to put together positive and negative feelings (in her pictures, for example, of the house), but this had not occurred in her feelings about her father. As we suggested in discussing reasons for her silence above, her feelings remained split, with an inability to express positive feelings about her father and, less clearly perhaps, an inability to express negative feelings towards her mother. This is obviously a large area to leave unresolved. The therapist's sense, nonetheless, was that this was not a workable therapeutic issue for Anna at this point, however much in theory it seemed desirable that she should resolve it, but that it might become more pressing over the next few years and, very probably, with puberty if not before. Anna's own capacity for development, together with her mother's relative openness, and what seemed to be her father's gradually increasing receptiveness, seemed hopeful signs that she would be able to resolve this when she was ready – and perhaps just as relevant, when her parents were able to allow her to do so. Perhaps this resolution would be achieved within Anna's current environment, the therapist mused, without the necessity for further therapeutic intervention.

THEORETICAL ISSUES

Children's responses to divorce

The number of children affected by divorce in Britain each year is estimated to be more than 170,000, double the figure for 1971. One child in five will experience their parents' divorce before the age of 16, and one in five school children live in single parent families or with only one of their birth parents. However, the fact that divorce is now so common may be misleading, and may even blind us to the fact that for the individual child the experience may be profoundly isolating and disturbing. Children must adjust to the separation from one parent, the formation of a new and different relationship with the other, changes in home and/or school and economic status, custody and contact battles, and different ways of living. Even where separation and divorce bring relief from conflict and anxiety, there are new circumstances and new relationships to be negotiated.

Recent research has begun to underline the difficulties many children experience as a result of their parents' separation (Cockett and Tripp, 1994), although the picture is complicated by the need to distinguish between the adverse consequences which result from conflict or other factors (such as financial difficulties), rather than from the divorce *per se*. Furthermore, the short- and long-term effects may vary. The short-term damage which divorce inflicts can be considerable, ranging from, for example, declining academic performance to impaired self-confidence and social relationships, and mild and more serious eating disorders. Although the research suggests that most children do recover and make successful re-adjustments, the predicted time span – two to three years – which this involves, takes a large amount of time out of any childhood or adolescence. Younger children appear to make a poorer overall adjustment to divorce than older children, and therefore may need greater understanding and help from adults. Ayalon and Flasher, for example, discuss how young children's more complete dependence on their parents make them 'very vulnerable to turbulence in the latter's lives' (1993: 5) and state that:

> Children up to the age of eight are especially vulnerable and often regress to behaviour characteristics of much younger children, such as crying, wetting, having sleeping problems and imaginary fears . . . They cling to adults and demand excessive approval and support. (1993: 25)

Nonetheless, as the story of Anna compared with her brother illustrates, children do respond very differently to the experience. Anna's difficulties in adjusting to her parents' separation demonstrates the importance of looking closely at a child's individual post-separation situation and, in particular, of examining the psychological meaning each parent has for each child. Current research on the effects of parental separation has been criticised as failing as yet to give us this kind of detailed picture of the child's response, and particularly does not do so from the child's own perspective (Healey et al., 1990). What the research does demonstrate is that children's and parents' reports of children's adjustment and changed parental relationships following separation tend to differ from one another (Kurdek et al., 1981; Healy et al., 1990). Anna's play therapy sessions support this: her play did show differences between her mother's interpretation of how Anna viewed her father's violence, which her mother saw as an attack on herself and not on the children, and Anna's own belief that the attack was a direct one on her and threatened her own safety.

Another factor in existing research is that it relies on children's verbal reports of their relationships with parents and their adjustment in order to arrive at the child's perspective. Yet Anna's case clearly demonstrates that non-verbal, 'play' communication was essential to help her in exploring and comprehending her internal state; of course, direct communications with her mother were also necessary to her. Non-directive play therapy, with its goal of facilitating the child's own exploration of his or her inner reality with minimal direction by the therapist, as Anna's case illustrates, can therefore be helpful in enabling us to understand more completely children's own perspectives on important life events such as divorce.

The utilisation of non-verbal methods to understand children's perspectives on crucial life events will be especially important with younger children who do not have the verbal and mental capacities required for completion of self-report measures. Anna's experiences, which can aid us in understanding features of other somewhat similar cases, seemed especially difficult for her, not only because of her young age, but also for the following reasons: her parents' conflicts strongly affected parent–child relationships; physical violence in the parental relationship was witnessed by the child; and the family system prior to separation may have been more dysfunctional than in many families.

Adjustment to their parents' separation seems to be much easier for children when parents manage to maintain joint, cooperative parental roles with their children, which are separate from their changed role to one another. The parents will then still be able to work together to meet their children's developmental needs (Ayalon and Flasher, 1993). For Anna and her brother, their parents were unable to work cooperatively on any level to meet their children's emotional and physical needs. This resulted in Anna's mother feeling overwhelmed by what she perceived as her sole responsibility for Anna's well-being, whereas previously she believed that some of Anna's needs were being met by her father. It is also possible that Anna was more anxious about a potential loss of her mother because she had already lost contact with her father by her parents' separation. As Ayalon and Flasher point out:

> Losing a parent by divorce inevitably raises the fear of losing the other one. The fear is so fierce that it can hardly be approached directly. (1933: 62)

Children's common fear of abandonment by the remaining parent seemed greatly compounded for Anna by the physical violence her mother experienced from her father and by Anna herself being a witness to this violence. Research on children who have witnessed repeated episodes of violence between their fathers and mothers at home have found that these children more frequently show symptoms of high distress and maladjustment than comparable children from non-violent families. Hurley and Jaffe (1990) and Jaffe et al. (1986) list a range of maladaptive behaviours in these affected children, such as sleep disturbances, aggression, poor concentration, passivity, hypervigilance, guilt and severe anxiety. These descriptions are very similar to other lists of symptoms compiled on children who have themselves been abused or traumatised, which has been recognised by Carroll. She concludes:

> Children who witness aggressive outbursts between their parents may be traumatized by the violent episodes themselves. (1994b: 10)

Unlike some traumatised children, Anna did not exhibit specific 'flashbulb' memories of these events nor did she seem to display behavioural re-enactments prior to her therapy (Pynoos and Eth, 1984, 1986; Terr, 1988; Hendricks et al., 1993). However, her sleep disturbance may have been directly related to the attacks on her mother, which occurred in the late evening, and to Anna's perceived need to remain hypervigilant at night to guard against further attacks. She seemed to feel unsafe inside her house in her own bed, partly perhaps because of the real events which had occurred in the night, and partly perhaps because she may have experienced persistent terrifying memories in her dreams, which she defended herself rigidly against in her waking life.

Other signs of trauma in her play therapy sessions were Anna's strongly expressed fearfulness and anxiety in the sessions themselves. In the early sessions Anna also seemed to show emotional numbing and denial of her negative emotions. She later began to express her negative feelings in her painting, making her house black, yet without dispensing with the positive feeling that it was more pleasant outside her house. Her drawing of the girl's distorted and black mouth in one of her paintings may also have been a symbolic means of expressing her trauma. It may have been related to Anna's identification with her mother, which she had demonstrated, for instance, in her play by dressing dolls and tidying up. The mouth may have represented the injuries about the mouth her mother was said to have received in one of her worst beatings. The distortion of the girl's mouth may also have depicted Anna's own feelings of sadness and terror, yet her total inability to articulate these emotions overtly or to deal with events which were frightening her. (See chapter 7, for a more extended discussion of this issue.)

Another reason for Anna's emotional difficulties may have been that the family itself for a long period prior to her parents' separation and her father's violence towards her mother was not meeting the children's and adults' needs. (As we indicated above, the research highlights the difficulty in general of distinguishing the adverse effects of conflict in the family from those arising from the separations of divorce itself.) Indications of this were Judith's complex feelings of guilt, dependence and responsibility towards her husband which seemed unrealistic. The patterns in Judith's responses to some extent resembled a 'victim' mentality, which battered and emotionally abused adults often begin to take on toward their abusers (see for example, the paradoxical phenomenon termed the 'Stockholm syndrome', Strenz, 1980; Bahn, 1980; Bettelheim, 1979). Judith's need for therapeutic help seemed due to her longstanding, dysfunctional relationship with Tom. The children also were affected by this because a family's marital relationship is '. . . the axis around which all other family relationships are formed' (Satir, 1967: 1). The children's relationships with their father appeared to have been polarised: Daniel seemed to have developed a role of emotional distance from his father; and Anna seemed to have been chosen by her father and mother to fulfil Tom's need for emotional closeness. Because the adult members in the family were not able to maintain an emotionally healthy relationship, the children's designated roles in the family would tend not to be appropriate for them and would not have fulfilled their developmental needs adequately.

Individual help or family conciliation

Because of Anna's individual situation, therefore, she experienced emotional difficulties in response to her parents' separation and required therapeutic help. Such referrals can sometimes present the therapist with a dilemma: the individual child is clearly experiencing distress but, equally clearly, this is as a result of the breakdown in the relationship between the couple, and, in Anna's case, the violence which has occurred between them. Ideally, individual therapeutic help would be offered in conjunction with some form of family conciliation aimed at helping the parents to resolve conflicts, particularly concerning questions of custody and contact, between them, and to reach agreements without resorting to the courts. Where agreements can be reached, the research suggests that these are more successful than ones which are imposed on the family by the courts. For the children, the experience of seeing parents who have been at loggerheads trying to resolve the issues between them amicably, can be extremely reassuring (Walker et al., 1994).

In Anna's case, the conflict between the couple was so extreme that there seemed a poor immediate prospect of involving them together in such a process. Sometimes, however, the therapist may need to consider, assuming the child needs individual help, whether to wait until some attempt at *rapprochement* has been made through conciliation. One of the dilemmas facing the therapist in Anna's case was that the approach to her for help had been made by Anna's mother, at the suggestion of her therapist. In these situations, it is always harder to ensure that the non-referring parent does not feel that the therapist too will be ranged against him/her in support of the other parent and child. S/he is likely to be the non-custodial parent and therefore in any case prone to feeling excluded from decision-making, and may well feel, as Anna's father did, that the therapist will have been recruited by 'the other side' and will have bought their story. It is not easy to reverse this message, once given and, although in Anna's case the therapist did manage to some extent to mollify her father, in our view, if it can be arranged some joint work between the couple before individual work is undertaken with the child is almost always preferable.

There has also been, within the developing field of conciliation services, disagreement about how children should be involved in the process, some services still preferring to see the children together with their parents, while others exclude them from the meetings altogether. The interested reader is referred elsewhere for a discussion of these issues (James and Wilson, 1986). However, our account of Anna's sessions illustrates the importance of non-verbal methods in facilitating an understanding of the child's perspective. Since conciliation as an approach is predominantly based on adult, verbal means of communicating, children may need other, non-verbal methods to express their needs and explore problems, as we have demonstrated here. (See also Wilson and Ryan, 1994a, for a discussion of the relative merits of using family therapy and individual approaches for children.)

Contact with the non-custodial parent

The final issue we consider is the complex question of Anna's future contact with her father. Every child needs to develop as realistic a picture as possible of each of their parents (Wolff, 1989), but this task is made more difficult for children after parental separation because of their tendency to form an alliance with one 'good parent' (Wallerstein and Kelly, 1980). This may at times be simply derived from the wish to reduce the complexity of their situation or from the wish to punish the parent who is no longer available on a daily basis.

There has, over the past three decades, been considerable disagreement in the research and professional literature over the question of contact between the non-custodial parent and the child. The case was prominently made by Goldstein et al. (1973) for contact to cease between them, where there continues to be conflict between the separated parents, on the grounds that the experience of continuing conflict between the parents was more damaging to the child than the loss of contact with one parent. Predictably, this view prompted disagreement, and a number of studies and discussion papers have examined children's different experiences of contact. Broadly speaking, the research suggests that children will make a healthier adjustment where they can remain in contact with both parents, where the level of conflict between the parents is low, and where the children themselves have some control over how and when they make contact with the non-custodial parent (Kelly, 1993).

This last issue is one which can create dilemmas for the adults involved, especially when, as with Anna, the child clearly expresses a wish not to see the other parent. Anna seemed to wish to banish her father, and this feeling was reflected in what she said to her mother. (We discuss further the issue of wish fulfilment in children's play, defences, motives and reality constraints, the child's developmental needs and the requirement of complete psychological information when making decisions for children's future in chapter 7 on assessments for court proceedings.) These difficulties were topics, among others, which the therapist would need to discuss with Judith in their meeting during Anna's later sessions. The therapist was also aware of American follow-up research on middle-class girls from divorced families (Wallerstein and Corbin, 1989) showing evidence of possible delayed reactions to divorce. Daughters who had developed close relationships to their mothers over their early adolescent period tended to identify with their mothers in their own adulthood. If their mothers had not developed a successful relationship subsequently, the daughters in turn found it more difficult to develop close intimate heterosexual relationships themselves, as well as having emotional difficulties in leaving their mothers on their own. The therapist intended to guide Judith toward these potentially difficult later transitions for Anna during their subsequent discussions.

However, Anna's story also highlights the difficulties of applying research findings rigidly to individual cases. In this case, the therapist considered, because of Anna's earlier, apparently good, relationship with her father, and based on her likely developmental needs, that ideally both parents should work together to restoring contact between father and daughter in the future. It was important that both parents move jointly towards a working relationship over Anna's needs. The therapist also considered that Anna's trauma at the violence between her parents had been great and that early contact with her father would rock her new sense of security if both parents had not sufficiently changed their own attitudes towards one another's trustworthiness regarding Anna. The therapist's opinion therefore was that this contact be temporarily postponed. Both parents needed nonetheless to be aware that, although postponing the renewal of contact might be in Anna's short-term interests, the possibility of renewing contact should, again in her interests, be kept under close review.

CONCLUSION

Parental separation and divorce do not necessarily cause lasting or serious emotional damage to every child, nor does each child need therapeutic help, as Anna's brother's case demonstrates. However, as we have noted, the period of adjustment to new patterns of relationships within the family may take a substantial period of time for a child. During this time a child will be more vulnerable to any additional major adjustments in his or her life, such as changes in school, financial status, or housing, which divorce often brings (Ayalon and Flasher, 1993). Any additional traumatic losses and severe family stresses may also trigger an emotional reaction in a child and may require therapeutic help.

Finally, the developmental changes in adolescence may entail increased vulnerability for a child. Learning and behavioural problems, and other more overt signs of emotional distress may develop at adolescence in a child who was very young during his or her parents' divorce, and who seemed to be making a good adjustment during middle childhood (Johnston and Campbell, 1988). As Wallerstein and Corbin's (1989) research highlights, adult relationships and independence may also be a period of increased stress. Carers and professionals should be aware of these potential areas of strain so that they can be alert to the need for practical and therapeutic responses towards children who as the result of parental separation and divorce may have heightened emotional vulnerability during the course of their development.

We turn in the next chapter to Delroy, whose emotional vulnerability seemed not only acute to his carers, social worker and therapist, but most distressingly of all, overwhelming to the child himself.

Chapter 5

Delroy
A Child Without Support

Children are dumb to say how hot the day is,
How hot the scent is of the summer rose,
How dreadful the black wastes of evening sky,
How dreadful the tall soldiers drumming by.
                                    Robert Graves

This is an account of twelve play therapy sessions, which were conducted over a six-week period with Delroy, a remarkably attractive eight year old, mixed race child with large wide-set dark brown eyes, full well-formed lips, high forehead and cheek bones and an Afro hair style. Remembering and writing about him has not been easy even now that some time has passed, because these recollections are tinged with the sadness of knowing that his life is not developing in a direction anyone would have wished for him. Five years on, he is still in the residential centre for children with epilepsy which he was waiting to attend when his play therapy began. There is still no sign of a family environment for him and realistically there is little chance of any successful family placement being found for him in the future. Reports from his residential centre show that, far from having made any emotional progress, his behaviour has deteriorated as he enters puberty. His behaviour has become increasingly sexualised, and he is now said to represent an acute danger to other children because of his aggressive attacks and calculated, devious sexual behaviour towards them. He masturbates openly, at times urinates on the floor, is self-destructive and is regarded as uneducable. His most recent report concludes that his placement is no longer suitable for him because of the danger that he now poses to other children. A transfer to a therapeutic community placement is being urgently considered.

Delroy's story is most certainly not a successful one, then. Nonetheless, we wanted to write about Delroy's sessions for three reasons. First, we recognise that all professionals working with troubled children will have children whose outcomes after their help seem worse rather than better. Sometimes an awareness of another professional's difficulties, such as those described here, can give a new perspective, leading to increased understanding of one's own experiences. It is often difficult – and supervision is important here – when emotionally 'failure' is writ large, for conscientious professionals to achieve a realistic balance between personal responsibility for that child's lack of progress, and feeling angered or becoming overwhelmed by other people and circumstances which have made the help offered ineffectual.

A second reason for including Delroy's story is that his narrative highlights the limitations of play therapy; that is, what therapy can and cannot do by way of change. During our therapeutic relationship it became very obvious that he needed dependable committed adults to nurture and be responsive to him – an attachment relationship, in other words – and that this need was so great that, without it, he found it difficult to engage fully in play therapy. This big gap in his life was evident at the outset. However, it was not until our sessions were under way that the dearth of even temporary attachments to adults in his current life really became clear. As will be apparent below, the instability of Delroy's emotional life made even very limited therapeutic goals unattainable.

A final reason for including Delroy's story is that his sessions illustrate the way in which a child's complex emotional issues readily emerge in play therapy which is non-directive. Delroy expressed troubled emotions related to his epilepsy in his sessions, but these difficulties were entangled with other emotional problems, which seemed to be more directly related to his traumatic experiences in earlier childhood, and perhaps to his disadvantaged status in society.

DELROY'S BACKGROUND

Delroy's social worker, Jane, began her account by describing his family history to me. He was the younger of two children; his older brother, Lee, was twelve years old and lived with their maternal grandmother. Their father, who was Afro-Caribbean, had left their mother several years ago, when Delroy was one year old. Jane believed their mother's only comment to her children about their father had been that he'd 'gone back to Jamaica'. Delroy had now been in foster care for six months, following an allegation he had made to his teacher about being sexually abused by his mother's partner, Ray. There had been no prosecution of the partner because of lack of evidence; Delroy's mother had dismissed the allegations and had been unwilling to have her partner leave home. To make the risk of further abuse to Delroy even greater, his mother had seen no reason to stop her partner from minding him after school while she continued to work full-time as a cleaner. In order to protect Delroy, the courts decided that he should be taken into care.

Delroy had already been under a court supervision order carried out by the local authority because of earlier serious problems in his relationship with his mother. His medical problems had obviously played a part in these. He had been diagnosed as having temporal lobe epilepsy at the age of two and had been on medication since then. There had been some difficulty initially in getting his mother to accept his need for daily medication; she chose instead to rely on homeopathic remedies. Even after accepting that Delroy must have his medication daily, she still found him very difficult to manage. Rather than giving him extra love and care, she tended to respond in kind to his outbursts of temper and foul language, punishing him severely for making her life more difficult by wetting the bed, and teasing him constantly about his 'babyish' ways. Equally worryingly, she had been unable to control his tendency as he got older to wander out of the house, which looked onto a busy road. Since Delroy had come into care, his mother had sold all the belongings he had left behind. This seemed to have been done more as a gesture of defiance towards the local authority than a rejection of Delroy, for she continued to turn up regularly for contact visits at his foster home, and certainly professed and continued to show affection for him.

Delroy's time in foster care had not been easy either. Three foster placements had broken down because his carers had found it too difficult to deal with his aggressive behaviour, to guard against his unpredictable flights from the house and to anticipate his seizures. Delroy's current short-term foster placement had been his longest yet. His carers, Mary and Gregory, had managed, just, to keep going with him, but the foster home had two other younger foster children in it together with the carers' own three teenage children. Mary and Gregory were struggling to meet the competing demands of all the children and were finding it virtually impossible to provide the large amount of individual attention Delroy needed.

The foster carers' situation was made even more difficult, Jane added, because Delroy's special school, which he had been attending on a daily basis, had just closed down. No other school had been sought because of the local authority's arrangement to send him to a residential treatment centre for children with epilepsy in the near future, with the aim of assessing his overall progress and establishing some management routines for his epilepsy. While he was waiting to go to the school, Delroy needed some space where he could look at his feelings of loss of his mother and the pending loss of his foster carers. Could I help?

After considering professional reports on Delroy and other professional information from his social services file, I decided that, although major changes in his functioning would be highly unlikely, given the precariousness of his placement, his serious emotional and physical problems and the short time scale available to us, play therapy sessions might provide him with an environment in which to deal with some of his current feelings. It might also relieve some of the heightened emotional pressure on his carers and on Jane, who all felt overwhelmed by his great need. These gains would probably offset the negative impact I anticipated of introducing myself, yet another adult, into his life on a short-term basis, at a time when his anxiety would already be heightened because of the impermanence of his care and his deteriorating physical condition.

I met with Mary, Gregory and Jane, and then had an introductory meeting with Delroy himself at his foster home. I proposed to see Delroy on a twice-weekly basis for his six remaining weeks with the carers. This twice-weekly arrangement partly reflected the shortness of time available to work in, and partly my judgement of Delroy's limited mental and emotional capacity, which would, I thought, make the usual once-weekly sessions too diluted to benefit him. Jane informed me that she intended to transport Delroy to his sessions herself, because of the foster carers' commitments at home. I questioned her decision, wanting his carers to be involved and also knowing her busy schedule, but Jane said she felt that it was important she took on this task. I asked that Mary or Gregory come for the first session at least.

DELROY'S PLAY THERAPY SESSIONS

Delroy's play therapy did not run smoothly, not only because, as we shall see, he challenged to the utmost my ability to set clear, firm limits, but also because of his desperate need for an attachment figure, an issue we shall explore more fully in our theoretical discussion at the end of the chapter. It became apparent that Delroy's strongest current attachment was to his social worker, Jane. His distress when she was unable to transport him to his session or when she went on holiday for a week, was sometimes extreme, and very debilitating for him in our sessions together. Despite these obstacles to his emotional relaxation, Delroy did work on a variety of personally important issues, including his need for physical closeness and physical safety, both of which seemed to be intimately linked to his epilepsy and to his earlier care. He also played out feelings more directly related to his earlier sexual abuse. We discuss his play therapy by considering six themes which emerged during his sessions.

First theme: Delroy's need for physical closeness and feelings of vulnerability

In the event, Jane had brought Delroy on her own, without his foster carers, for his first session. As soon as Jane left, promising to return,

Delroy came close up to me and hugged me, then remained standing very near me. His sudden affectionate behaviour took me rather by surprise, but I contained my spontaneous response and said, 'You don't know me very well, but you want to be near me'. I turned on the audiotape, explaining what I was doing, even though Delroy seemed uninterested in my action or words. He seemed more concerned about positioning himself very close to me again and staring at me. 'You have to have a good look at me because you don't know me', I said. He smiled, and started to fiddle with the rings on the finger of my left hand, thus curtailing my hand movements.

I immediately sensed in a direct personal way that physical closeness was unusually important for Delroy. I had an atypical strong surge of feeling smothered by his physical presence. However, repeated comments on his overly familiar behaviour did not seem appropriate to me in these first few minutes of our first session. Instead, I wanted him to feel accepted by me. Delroy continued to stand leaning against my side and I said gently that I was going to sit down. As I gradually moved towards the chair, Delroy asked rather uneasily where Jane was. I replied factually that Jane had told us that she was going to the shops across the road, and then would come back and wait for him, adding that maybe he was feeling a bit strange here with me and wished Jane was near him. Delroy's response was to move quickly towards me as I talked and to stand holding on to my arm as I finished. 'Maybe you want to be near me when Jane is gone.' Delroy said, 'yes'. I added, 'You need somebody big to be near you and take care of you'. Delroy did not seem to listen, being in the process of rapidly releasing my arm and going over to pick up the play clock.

Delroy's need for physical contact was frequently apparent in his play and his interactions with me, and this theme was strongly evident from our first session onwards. For example, he would touch my face as if feeling my responses or mood; he would touch the hands of the clock as he tried to master the numbers; and when later he began to use paints and papers to draw, he would touch the object as if needing to feel its shape as he drew it.

His sense of physical vulnerability also emerged in a recurrent play sequence involving farm animals. For example, in his second session, he put together a big fence for the large animals and another separate one for the little ones, which he placed inside the fence. Delroy became increasingly perturbed when he could not manage to get all of the small horses to stand upright. 'You think it's important, Delroy, that the little ones don't fall over. I could help.' Delroy ignored my offer, but seemed to console himself by saying that they would be asleep soon.

I said: 'Yes, Delroy, then they can't fall down and get hurt. They'll be lying down asleep and safe.' He then picked up all the animals and crowded them into the doll's house (reminding me irresistibly of all the people I saw metaphorically squeezing into his foster carer's three-bedroomed council house when I had visited). Delroy again repeatedly tried to get all the horses to stand up, telling me in a serious tone of voice, 'We don't want them to wobble any more.' 'You get very worried and want to help them when they wobble. Maybe we both could help to stand them up.' Delroy ignored my offer of help.

Delroy returned to this play sequence in his later sessions, seemingly to have progressed somewhat in his trust of me. He was now able to interact with me. Delroy settled down to playing with the horses once again, sharing a few this time with me. We both had a selection of white, brown and black ones. He made a playdough cover for his horses, then put a cover over mine, making sure that the legs of mine, which were showing, were covered up. I commented that now the horses were covered, warm – maybe I should have said 'safe' or 'cosy', or 'hidden away', only I wasn't sure what this represented. He gave me yet more playdough for my horses to eat as he fed his own, and I said, 'You want to take care of my horses as well'. He produced a big horse from his own collection and asked me whether I wanted it, and I replied, 'You want to be kind to me, giving me your big one'.

He carefully propped the animals up, then commented that they were falling down, propped them up again, and repeated this two or three times, quite intensely. I reflected his feeling of worry when they fell over, needing help to stand up, maybe worried that they would get hurt. Delroy nodded vehemently at these remarks.

In a later session he again played with the animals, which seemed to me to reflect his need for physical safety. Delroy got out the farm animals and began covering them in the sand, and making a wall to go round them. He found this difficult, but persisted, then arranged the animals carefully inside, making sure, by taking my hand and putting it underneath the horses, that I caught them if they wobbled or looked unsafe. When I did this, I said things like, 'You want me to catch it. If it falls, I can catch it. It goes in my hand. It feels safe.' We sat together by the sand, side by side. Delroy turned and gave me a hug, which felt like a warm, unforced embrace. I returned his hug easily, saying that he was feeling happy with me.

Second theme: sexual abuse

Some of Delroy's play sequences during his play therapy sessions seemed to help him rework experiences which had been sexually abusive, supporting and amplifying the allegations he had made before his sessions began. Jane telephoned just before Delroy's fifth session to say that Delroy had earlier alleged sexual abuse by Ray, his mother's cohabitee, and also by a man, Jerry, at the special school he attended. He had talked to his foster carer about it being nice when he was at home, being cuddled by Ray in bed. He was also specific about Jerry touching his penis and that he had touched Jerry's penis. Jane had notified the police and would be going with Delroy to a joint investigation later in the day, but meanwhile Delroy was carrying on 'as normal' and would see me at the usual time.

In the session that followed these allegations, Delroy went to the tray, took some scissors, and began cutting the paper into a long ribbon. I commented that it was maybe like a snake, but got no response from Delroy, who went on quietly cutting, not looking at me. I focused on what he was doing and said, 'You're making it longer and longer', then, after a moment, seeing his hands drooping, 'You seem tired today'. Delroy said, very definitely and surely, 'I'm not tired', continued to cut, and then went and got out the water pump and pushed it hard up and down several times. He came and sat on the bean bag, but slipped off on to the floor and looked worried though not hurt. I reflected these feelings as Delroy came near me. He leant into me, took the pump, put it on my head and laughed. I said, 'You think I look silly', and he came closer and hugged me to his chest.

My face was in his chest and I could feel that he had taken the pump off my head and was resting his chin very hard on my head. I could feel him putting the pump on my head again, rubbing my head. He said, laughing gleefully and loudly, 'You're liking it'. I said, 'I'm not sure what you're doing; I'm feeling a bit squashed. It's exciting for you', I added, as Delroy laughed again, then looking at the clock, asked what time it was. I told him, he released me, brought his chair to face me as I sat on the bean bag, and thrust the pump into my ear, then sat back and looked at me expectantly.

I said, 'That felt strange. You're waiting to see what I do. I didn't know what to do.' Delroy, laughing with excitement, came around behind me, trying to get the pump under my skirt. I said, 'No Delroy, you can't do that to me. It's a private place for me.' He quickly put the pump on to my shoe, and laughed again, then went back to the table and hung his head down towards the floor, not looking at me or saying anything for some time. Then he said, 'You put away the pump'. As I did so, I commented 'You don't want to touch the pump; you want me to help you get rid of it'. And then added, 'You seem sad now, maybe not sure you can talk to me after doing all those things. But I didn't let you do anything that was bad. Maybe you were thinking of things that happened to you, that were not playing, but were real things and naughty. But you didn't know how to stop them.' Delroy listened quietly, not looking at me, but very alert.

It seemed likely that other sequences, too, of behaviour during his sessions involved echoes for him of his experiences of sexual abuse. For example, in an early session, he showed a marked speed and lack of selfconsciousness in removing his shorts to try on a cowboy outfit, despite my telling him to put them on again, seemingly unaware of the inappropriateness of remaining undressed in the playroom. This was quickly followed by an episode of play in which, in the process of putting the little animals inside their fence, Delroy chewed on the tail of a small white horse. He commented that the little one had to go 'there'. 'If it was with the big ones, its tail would get bitten off.' I replied, 'The little white one's very afraid of getting his tail hurt by the big ones. You're making sure it's safe and not hurt.' (I thought to myself how this remark fitted the classic use of sexual symbolism, in Freud's Little Hans, but guarded myself against an over-reaction with Delroy due to my own associations.)

This episode, with its possible sexual connotations, may have been triggered for him by his removal of his clothes and my request that he should keep his clothes on. In both these incidents, my responses remained within the metaphor used by Delroy, and attempted to clarify for him feelings of excitement which were intermingled with heightened anxiety.

Third theme: the need for adult approval

The experience of sexual abuse and perhaps Delroy's underlying feeling of being a 'burden' to others, increased by his disability, his racial identity and his time in foster care, would also explain another theme which emerged in his therapy and behaviour: namely that he tried at times desperately to please adults. He would give inappropriate affectionate responses, such as kisses and hugs, to adults he had just met, as we saw above in his initial greeting of me, and as I observed on occasion when he would leave the playroom and greet total strangers in the waiting room with a hug. Delroy also seemed to block out any negative feelings he might have towards adults, or they might have towards him, as being too threatening. For example, when our hour had ended, as on occasion it did, with a struggle over Delroy wanting more time, he seemed in the ensuing session to try and propitiate me.

In the third session, when he showed me the new shoes and a blue jersey he had on, he seemed to be trying very hard to get positive attention from me (we had had a struggle over his leaving last time). I reflected his feeling of wanting me to like him and think he looked nice.

Delroy then began a card game, with rules (very simple) made up by him and, as we played the game, he commented that he had played with the marbles last time. I said, 'Yes, the marbles are important to you.'

    D: I wanted 'em.
    V: Yes, and you were cross with me. I said they had to stay here. Then you gave them back to me. Now they're back in here, like I said.

Delroy went back to the cards and kept smiling. He started holding my hand firmly, and persisted in pulling my hand to his face. I allowed Delroy to do this, saying, 'You want me to like you. You want me to touch your face, to show you I like you', as I smiled at him. (I was conscious that I couldn't just smile at him to be nice, that he needed me to touch him, too.)

At the beginning of his eighth session (after another difficulty about leaving), Delroy seemed rather subdued and worried, then began drawing around stencils, giving me hugs and smiling a good deal. At the second hug I said, 'You're not cross with me today. Maybe you're remembering you were very cross with me last time, and I got worried about you as well.' Delroy said, 'Yes', and sighed. 'We didn't have a very good time together.' 'No. Next time when I come it will be nice.' 'Maybe you can't *always* be nice when you're upset.' 'No.' Delroy laughed. 'You try to be kind, but sometimes you're cross, aren't you?' Delroy hugged me again.

    V: You're trying to make up for it now. You don't like getting cross with me. People don't like being cross.
    D: [changing the subject] The sun's going in your eyes. Over there.

He put his hand on my face to protect my eyes from the sun, judging precisely where to put his hand.

    V: You're guarding it. Being kind.
    D: Look, the sun's not there any more.

Fourth theme: Delroy's cognitive and mental development

I was initially disconcerted to discover the severity of Delroy's condition, and his poor cognitive functioning. His referral information had not prepared mr adequately for its extent. For example, in his first session, when explaining that we would see each other in the playroom and stop when he went to his new school to live, Delroy responded by asking whether I had been in the car with them, evidently unable to remember who had been with him in the car on a visit the day before to his new school. It quickly became obvious that Delroy's emotional and cognitive development was limited, and that his limitations were magnified both by physical and emotional causes. Thus the vagueness, which to some extent was attributable to his epilepsy, also became far worse under stressful conditions.

Delroy's limited mental development meant that my non-verbal signals, similarly to working with a younger child (such as Patrick) had to be vividly and very easily communicated. Thus I deliberately mimicked Delroy's frowns and grimaces of distaste to convey my meaning to him more easily. I was also aware that responses to him needed to be couched in simple language, to be repeated sometimes several times over and, if necessary, persistently. At the end of each session, I had, for example, not only to alert him to the time, as one would with any child, but also to show him this repeatedly and in detail on the clock. Dates on the calendar also had to be shown to him repeatedly, so that he could begin to get some internal sense of time passing from visualising it in a concrete way. By the end of the sessions he had made some small progress in mastering telling the time and understanding when he would be coming again.

In the card games which Delroy played periodically, it was evident that he could not operate with even simple rules for very long, and had poor concentration and memory in these situations. His sudden mood changes and distractibility also seemed more typical of a much younger child. Again, during the sessions, he made some small progress in memorising and concentrating, for example, in painting or in playing these card games. It was also, however, notable that in other sequences of play, such as one he had devised involving trains on a track, he did have the capacity to concentrate for considerable lengths of time and also seemed more highly engaged emotionally.

Delroy's immature development was evident in his lack of inhibition, for example, his unselfconsciousness in taking off his shorts suggested the behaviour of a much younger child. He also had difficulty establishing his own routines (see chapter 2 on Patrick), so that, for example, ending each session was clearly difficult for him. It seemed likely that this difficulty stemmed from multiple reasons associated with attachment and fears arising from a lack of dependent adults (if no one is there, then I can trust only myself) which are particularly critical for a child with a disability, as well as cognitive difficulties to do with understanding time. His difficulty in ending was probably more marked during his sessions because there were often changes in personnel coming to collect him.

For example, in one of his middle sessions, I warned him as usual ten minutes before the session ended that it would soon be time to stop. He turned away and busied himself further with the fences. I waited a few minutes, then remarked that Delroy was suddenly very busy and not wanting to listen to me. I followed this comment shortly by, 'It's time to go. You don't want to be finished.' Repeating 'it's time to go', Delroy first asked me to allow him to take the fences and marbles home with him. I refused, saying I needed him to leave everything: the marbles had to stay here too. He begged me in a whining, wheedling tone to take the marbles, just the marbles, for Mary to see. I again refused, acknowledging that maybe he thought I was being mean to him, but I wasn't. I liked him, but everyone left the toys here. He defiantly turned away from me to face the wall, ignoring me as I said that he had to leave everything here for other children to use, too. 'You're angry with me. You want to be special.' I paused, then repeated to him that none of the children took things away with them. I said firmly, 'You don't want to put them away, but you have to. Put the marbles back for next time.' 'No.' 'You like them, but you need to put them back . . . You're cross with me, but you still have to leave them.' Delroy continued scowling at me, and looking very cross, saying, 'No' loudly and angrily when I suggested I take them.

I said, 'I'm going to have them. It's a rule. I'm not trying to be mean and I'm not angry with you.' A long pause, while Delroy stood glaring at me. 'You're very cross with me. You want to be the boss. You want to make me give you the marbles, but I can't let you have them, they're not mine. All the children who come here need to play with them . . . I'm going now, Delroy. Time to go.'

I added that he could bring the marbles downstairs to show his driver this time, but then he had to give them back to me to take upstairs for next time (hoping to deflect him from a direct confrontation). Delroy left the room, saying nothing and looking straight ahead. But downstairs, Delroy easily talked to the volunteer driver, who had come to take Delroy home because Jane has been called to court. Delroy chatted to the driver about the marbles, and explained how he had wanted to bring the marbles home. Then when I reached out my hand for them, he handed them over quite easily. He smiled up at me and I returned a smile of goodbye, trying to match his now friendly and relaxed manner with me.

I thus responded to Delroy's reluctance to leave by trying to bring the experience more under his control, and letting him carry the marbles down to show the driver, while at the same time firmly maintaining the boundary on the play materials. In later sessions, Delroy still found it difficult to leave the playroom and the things in it, but seemed to be beginning to be able to reach the decision to do so himself, saying he would leave them, and play with them next time.

This progress was not, as one would expect over a critical emotional issue, unimpeded. For example, at the end of the eighth session, he accepted that he would leave the toys, but return next time and play with them – 'When I come back, I'll play' – and showed the beginnings of being able to use a coping mechanism for himself. However, two sessions later he took an item from the playroom (perhaps connected with his understanding that he would be ending his sessions soon), deftly concealing it beneath his jersey while my back was turned. I remembered his swift movement, caught from the corner of my eye, when I failed to find the blue jug Delroy had been playing with before he left. At the beginning of the next session, I asked him to return it, clearly restating the rule that toys had to remain in the playroom, but also acknowledging the feelings which had prompted him to take them.

> V: There's something I have to ask you, Delroy. Last time after you left, I couldn't find the little blue jug. I think you put it in your hand and took it home with you. You liked it so much, you wanted to keep it. You need to bring it back for me next time. You can put it in your coat pocket and bring it to play with here.

I thus tried to help him make his actions less emotionally loaded and secret. In the last two sessions, he seemed again to have re-established some inner controls, directing me to tidy the room later and seeming able to accept leaving.

This example also suggests that Delroy's moral development had not reached the level of developing internal controls himself on these actions or of feeling guilty for his actions. Delroy most probably felt ashamed and 'naughty', as he had in other instances during his sessions. He seemed to need adults in close proximity to impose their own rules of right and wrong consistently, as would a very young child (Kohlberg, 1976). His moral development had been distorted and delayed most probably not just by delay due to his physical impairment, or even his impairment in combination with his sexual abuse, which can lead to favours and gifts when the child 'pleases' the adult sexually, but also by his lack of an available, reassuring and firmly consistent attachment figure as he developed.

Fifth theme: setting appropriate limits

Delroy's moral development was part of the larger issue for Delroy of establishing therapeutic limits to his behaviour. Setting these appropriately, while at the same time acknowledging his right to feel in a particular way, was one of the key themes in Delroy's play therapy.

In general I needed to judge when it was necessary to exercise control myself, when to modify this partially, and when Delroy could be left to find and experience a limit himself. Following one session when Delroy slipped off down the stairs and out of the building, without heeding possible dangers from the busy road, I realised that I needed to set firmer limits myself. If necessary, I would to do this by physically controlling Delroy, particularly outside the playroom when he was most easily distracted and, when near the outer door, in most danger. However, I continued to help Delroy to work on this issue for himself, for example, by repeating the fact that he had the option to go to the playroom or to leave with the driver, but not to go into the other offices.

Another example was at the beginning of the ninth session, when Delroy seemed reluctant to come up and didn't want the volunteer driver, Roger, to leave. 'I asked Roger if he could stay, but he couldn't', I said to Delroy, as we stood in the hallway and as he was developing the recalcitrant look that he'd had when Jane left him other times, 'You don't like people to leave you'. I then gave him the choice either to come up to the playroom, or have the driver take him back to Mary's. I gave this choice to Delroy about three times and he finally decided to come up. 'You decided to go up. You feel safe with me', I said, at which Delroy gave me a huge, tight hug and a beaming smile.

Delroy's learning of basic limits to his behaviour in the playroom and his increasing understanding of the freedoms he did have within the playroom became more evident in his last two sessions. For example, he wanted to take the gun to show Mary, but seemed to accept it when I said that the things had to stay in the playroom, for him and for the other children. He remarked, as he left, 'When I come back, right, I'll play'. 'All the things will be here for you to play with', I replied.

He thus was beginning to be both able to direct me and to comply with my basic rules appropriately, albeit on a very rudimentary developmental level.

Delroy's need for my limit-setting also extended to behaviours which he had developed because of his sexual abuse. We discuss elsewhere therapeutic responses to children's sexualised behaviour and the ways in which the non-directive therapist allows the child to move from more distant symbolic expressions to more direct ones and then, perhaps to indirect ones again. With Delroy's sexualised responses to me during our fifth session, I did not directly interpret what he was doing in terms of its probable meaning, but reflected both his feelings, 'you're excited', and my own of feeling squashed and not knowing what to do in my probable role of the abused child. I also set an important limit for him, by stating that he should not put the pump under my skirt because that was private to me and he was not allowed to do so. I thus responded congruently, drawing on my own feelings of discomfort to give an appropriately healthy adult response to a child, but at the same time helping Delroy to be aware of his own feelings of arousal.

Later, when Delroy was clearly feeling discomforted and abashed, I pointed out that he had done nothing wrong, but that perhaps he had been thinking of things which had been done to him, which were wrong and which he had been unable to stop. This was said in a tentative way which I hoped would allow Delroy to listen and absorb, or reject my comments as he wished.

Sixth theme: Delroy's attachment needs

However, the theme which most coloured Delroy's therapy was his urgent attachment need. As we have indicated, in the absence of a more appropriate attachment figure, he had become dependent on his social worker, Jane, and his anxieties when she was not available or was going away were extreme, and left him unable to engage productively in his therapy sessions. This was most apparent in Delroy's seventh session, to which Jane brought him, explaining that she would be away for two weeks, and that a volunteer driver would bring him during this time.

Delroy went upstairs slowly, and lingered at the windows on the stairs, looking for Jane's car. I said that he didn't want Jane to leave, that he was sad to see her go. I asked him to go up, as he was still lingering, and he looked very cross. He said vehemently, 'I love Jane', and I said that he'd rather be with Jane than with me, that he was upset because Jane was going on holiday. Delroy turned on the stairs and ran down, trying to go out of the building. I said that he could go upstairs, or would have to sit on the chairs on the landing. He sat on one chair and I sat next to him, feeling uncomfortable in my conflicting role of both guarding him and being close to him. He chewed on a piece of cord from his jacket hood and glowered at me, and I tried to reflect his feelings: that he was cross with me, liked to chew when he was unhappy, 'maybe cross with Jane'. Delroy said vehemently at this that he was *not* cross with Jane. (This was too much for him to admit at this point, and an overinterpretation on my part.) He put his jacket over his head and I said that it was dark inside, and he was by himself, being unhappy. He turned to me for a moment, laughing slightly in a forced way, but when I said that he was trying to laugh, he began to glower again, and then got off the chair and started to kick the door, blocking the main doorway. I said that he wanted me to be cross with him, then we would both feel the same, but even though I knew he was unhappy, I was not cross. (But I *was* uncomfortable at this point, being aware that we were being disruptive. I regretted later keeping on doggedly.)

We spent several minutes on the landing, with a few people coming and going, and Delroy sitting in a corner on the floor with his foot blocking the door. I finally said that Delroy might rather be at Mary's, but he told me that Mary was out shopping. I then said that Delroy could go upstairs to the playroom if he wanted to, or I would phone for him to be taken back; when he nodded at my second suggestion, I telephoned Jane's office. As we waited, Delroy kept darting away into the other offices to peer closely at the secretaries. He went out to the waiting room, then suddenly bolted through the inner door towards the outside door. I was worried that he would run into the busy road, and took his arm at the entrance, saying, 'Come back', at which Delroy shouted 'Get off'. Turning his back on me he looked out of the window while I kept guard, putting my knee on his chair to prevent it tipping into the window. We remained like this for about 10 or 15 minutes, then Delroy announced that he had seen Jane's car, and slipped out of the door. He became extremely angry with me as we stood by the road, telling me to 'get off' as I held him firmly, fearing that he would hurl himself into busy traffic. Eventually, Jane arrived, and crossed the road to Delroy, who held her hand and stood there looking very subdued and small next to her. I said that Delroy was very upset and wanted so much just to be with Jane.

Jane told me over the telephone that Delroy had insisted that she spend the whole afternoon with him at his tutoring session. Jane had given him a tape to return to her after her holiday, and a calendar with the days to mark off. Roger, the volunteer driver, would call to see if he wanted to come to his play therapy session next week.

THEORETICAL ISSUES

Attachment issues within a play therapy context

The two dominant features of Delroy's personality and behaviour were his lack of attachment, and his emotional and intellectual immaturity, which seemed to arise in part from his medical condition of epilepsy, and in part from the emotional and physical neglect by his mother and the sexual abuse he had experienced earlier. Because these affected the conduct of his play therapy so clearly, we shall consider them first, together with issues which were raised by Delroy's emotional neediness concerning the limitations and timing of therapy.

Of the theories relevant to understanding Delroy's behaviour and needs, that of attachment seems to offer the best 'fit', and to help most in making sense of the dominant themes in his interaction with adults who were caring for him. 'Attachment', the term used to describe the tie which children develop with a preferred adult (usually a parent who has the main responsibility for looking after them) from about half way through the first year is distinguished from 'attachment behaviour', which is the outward manifestation of this tie, defined by Bowlby (1982) as 'seeking and maintaining proximity to another individual'.

According to Bowlby, this attachment behaviour begins to be clearly evident by about seven months, and is then exhibited readily and regularly until the end of the child's third year. The child begins to protest and become upset if separated from the familiar caregiver, and seeks closeness when frightened, upset or in a strange situation. As long as the child knows that the caregiver is nearby and can check this from time to time, he or she feels free to explore and can thus develop skills and independence. This stable relationship also helps the child to discover a sure sense of identity, both because of the responsiveness and acknowledgement of individual needs, and also because this stability enables the child to make new discoveries, and interact safely in other situations, without anxiety overwhelming these discoveries. Thus, in the developing child, the attachment system and the exploratory system which go to make up the self, are closely linked. However, when the child feels threatened, the attachment system is activated and the child's capacity to engage in other activities is reduced or rendered non-existent (depending on the degree of activation and the coping mechanisms of the child) until the attachment needs are met.

The attachment figure remains important throughout childhood as a base from which to explore the outside world and to which to retreat, but attachment behaviour is less obvious in the older child when attachment is felt to be secure. The need for attachment remains throughout life but, although attachment behaviour continues to be heightened at times of illness, the birth of a child, or other crises, it normally continues at a low level during adulthood. As this suggests, however, there are certain conditions or events, either within the child or in the environment, which are likely to produce heightened attachment behaviour, particularly in children. These include hunger, pain, ill health, rebuffs by other children or adults, fear, and certain behaviours on the part of the attachment figure, such as discouraging closeness, or departure.

When they are separated from their attachment figures for a prolonged time, children may react in different ways, either exhibiting a form of anxious clinging to an alternative attachment figure or appearing highly ambivalent, or becoming compulsively independent and detached.

Delroy seemed during his play therapy to be at an important point psychologically. He had not yet so despaired of forming attachments to parent figures that he had become apathetic and detached. On the contrary, he seemed desperately to be trying to form close attachments, but because of the absence of appropriate parent figures towards whom he could direct his feelings, he expressed his feeling indiscriminately, trying to get positive acknowledgement from any adult whom he encountered, regardless of the circumstances or their lack of response to him. His mother did not fulfil his attachment needs, either currently or, it appears, during his earlier life with her. Therefore, Delroy did not appear to have, as some children might, experience of a secure attachment relationship to transfer over to new carers. His circumstances in foster care also prevented him from beginning to develop a secure attachment, as, it appears, did his next placement. His most stable adult presence in his life at the time of his sessions, and the one that he seemed to have formed the closest attachment to, was his social worker, Jane. For obvious reasons, this could never fully meet his needs, and hence his anxieties when she was not there were extreme (whereas with a more consistently available attachment figure he might have been less distraught and able to transfer temporarily to another in her absence). As the narrative in the first part of this chapter shows, his desperation just before Jane went away on holiday was extreme. He became too engulfed with feelings about her leaving to be able to engage in his play therapy session and needed to spend time close to her in order to prepare himself for her departure. In addition, although by this time the therapist and the setting were familiar, the reflection of his troubled emotions in the sessions would also serve to heighten Delroy's emotional need for a secure base, as our theoretical understanding of the conditions which produce heightened attachment behaviour suggests. Thus, when this base was about to be removed from him, the demands of therapy became intolerable for him.

A further factor likely to make his need for an attachment relationship more acute was his physical ill-health. It is a commonplace clinical observation that children who are ill become more dependent and turn to an attachment figure with more frequency (Bowlby, 1979). Delroy's play sequences suggested that he was aware of himself as someone who needed more care than other children and that he felt more vulnerable to harm. His play involving the horses which he tried repeatedly to stand up when they fell down, conveyed vividly worries about falling and getting hurt without anyone to catch him. Thus a heightened, and realistic, sense of needing protection and care strengthened his normal need for a stable relationship with an adult.

Although the therapist was conscious of the importance of this attachment relationship for him, the precariousness of his other relationships and the level of his need for a secure base was not so apparent at the time of his referral as it became during the course of therapy. From this, two things clearly emerged.

First, Delroy's need for an attachment figure dominated much of his behaviour. As the model suggests, the fact that he was still actively trying to form an attachment was a positive sign of his openness to the possibility of a normal attachment relationship. However, it also meant that he was unlikely to make progress on other fronts, in particular in his intellectual development, while his attachment needs remained unmet. The therapist was therefore concerned, having seen the depth of his emotional needs, at the prospect of his being placed in a residential establishment, which because of the way it was staffed and organised, would be less likely to meet adequately his attachment needs.

Second, Delroy's experience of therapy raised questions about whether or not it was right to offer him play therapy at this point in his life. Clearly, with hindsight, his unmet attachment needs made play therapy largely ineffectual, and perhaps even at times compounded his distress.

A child's attachment needs then, are, in our opinion, of paramount importance, and may in certain circumstances, as in Delroy's case, make therapy ineffective. For some children, however, it seems clear that despite stable, potentially permanent placements with responsive caregivers, they are unable to develop close relationships without help. Their earlier experiences of non-existent or damaging attachment relationships suggests that the 'defensive seclusion', which they have developed as a protective shield against further pain prevents them from forming attachments to new parent figures, even when these are loving, responsive and available. In these cases an intensive therapeutic programme needs to be developed for the child which recognises the severity of his needs and helps him gradually overcome his difficulties (Fahlberg, 1986).

A related issue is that in the absence of suitable parent figures for the child, professionals may find themselves taking on more of a caregiving role than would usually be seen as appropriate. We consider this in our section, below, on personal issues for the therapist.

Delroy's emotional and intellectual impairment and its links with epilepsy

As we suggested earlier, emotional and physiological factors can be closely linked, and it may be impossible to disentangle completely the different effects within the child's behaviour.

We do not propose here to consider the complex differential diagnosis which can be made concerning epilepsy, although we would stress that in any therapeutic work it is important to clarify the nature of the diagnosis. In Delroy's case, for example, it would have been critical to know the extent to which the causes of Delroy's developmental delay were physiological. It was also relevant to consider what is known about the correlation between emotional disturbance and epilepsy which we sketch out below.

An epileptic seizure (Hopkins, 1984) is a kind of short-circuiting of the brain, in which an electrical discharge within the brain gives rise to movement, feelings or thoughts unrelated to the external situation. The outward manifestations of seizures depend on the site of involvement, the most common type being grand mal epilepsy (Taylor, 1982). Complex partial seizure, the form of epilepsy from which Delroy suffered, is more commonly known as temporal lobe epilepsy, and is characterised by unprovoked, episodic behavioural changes, a trance-like appearance, and on–off shifts in consciousness or perception, typically passing through four stages. The person experiencing the seizure may feel as if he or she were in a dream, may feel a sense of familiarity so that a situation experienced for the first time seems as if it is the recurrence of a past situation; objects may seem far away and small, or the opposite, close at hand and gigantic; sounds may become extremely muted or very loud; the person's body may feel distorted; the experience of foul smells are particularly common, often described as the smell of rotting eggs or burning rubber; and powerful feelings may erupt – feelings such as fear, loneliness, sadness or anger. This first phase usually lasts only a matter of seconds and is immediately followed by a second phase which is characterized by a loss of awareness, often manifested in a blank stare, or confused repetitive sounds. The third phase is the longest, persisting for some minutes and in exceptional cases for hours, the primary manifestation being automaton like behaviour, with jerky movements of neck and face. The fourth phase is a gradual transition over several minutes in which consciousness returns, the person feels groggy, and emerges often with little memory of what has gone before.

The person with epilepsy has recurrent, often widespread, transient disturbances of brain function but there is some disagreement as to the extent to which this results in brain damage. It has been stated (Gastaut, 1976) that there is associated brain damage, varying from the trivial to the incapacitating, in 95% of all epileptics. However, studies of intelligence in patients with epilepsy run into difficulties, not only because the populations studied may not be representative of the group as a whole, being largely drawn from residential and specialist centres, but also because the effects of medication may influence the results. Early age of onset, such as Delroy's, carries a poorer prognosis for mental functioning (Lennox and Lennox, 1960), and personality disorders are found more frequently the earlier the seizures start and the more widespread the convulsions.

Children with epilepsy have a much higher rate of psychiatric disorder than healthy children and than children with other chronic illnesses. Research suggests that several factors are associated with this increased vulnerability, including the type of neurological lesion, the individual characteristics of the child, and the disturbance or otherwise in other family members (Hoare, 1987). Finally, it is important not to lose sight of the stigma and hostility which those suffering from epilepsy often experience.

A number of factors emerged, as we have seen, in Delroy's therapy which were indicative of immature mental development, but seemed to be attributable both to his medical condition and to emotional difficulties. Thus, for example, his difficulty in picking up spatial clues was one feature of his behaviour in which the intricate relationship between emotional problems and physiological difficulties became apparent. His need to be physically close to the therapist, which came as such a surprise in the opening minutes of the first session, seemed to rise in part from the need to experience something through touch before he could fully understand it. It may also relate to his need to feel that an adult would be near at hand in case he had a fit. However, as we have already suggested, a child who is anxious about being able to keep contact with a dependable adult is likely also to become extra clingy in order to keep the adult from going away. So attachment behaviour, which one would expect to be heightened at the beginning of therapy, would be further strengthened by his cognitive limitations and his physical impairment.

The interlocking of emotional and intellectual features was also evident in Delroy's varying ability to concentrate on an activity for any length of time. In view of his difficulties in telling the time, or remembering rules or information, his capacity for long periods of concentration on a particular activity or sequence of play was very noticeable, and suggested the capability for educational progress. Equally, at other times he seemed unable to concentrate, and to become easily distracted, forgetful and vague about events.

Delroy's difficulty in managing to leave the play therapy room also seemed to have a physiological and an emotional component. In terms of attachment theory, it was as if he had little experience of a secure base from which to make forays into the world outside, having lacked the kind of sensitive caregiving which would gradually have enabled him to test out the safety of leaving his attachment figure over longer and longer distances (Taylor, 1971). However, it seemed possible that his epilepsy had also impaired his ability to pick up and use spatial clues, so that when he emerged from inside out into the street he felt completely without boundaries, and could not adapt to the physical space and use the normal indicators which a child of his age would usually respond to.

The interrelationship between different emotional and physical factors is a familiar feature of any assessment, particularly those involving children with a physical disability or illness. It becomes critical to maintain an awareness of the different aspects of a problem, and probably to try and develop some hierarchy of needs, when issues of the kind of care or treatment the child requires are involved. In Delroy's case, the decision was taken to make his medical needs paramount, and the need to stabilise his medication. The therapist's assessment of his emotional needs suggested that this would prove inadequate unless these were given primacy; sadly his current problems suggest that this was correct.

PRACTICE ISSUES

Race, gender and power within play therapy

All therapy by its nature involves some imbalance of power, in that embarking on it the client hands over, more or less willingly, some control of his fate to the therapist. In therapy with children, the power imbalance is arguably always greater: not only does the normal difference between adult and child exist, but also, the decision to refer the child, however carefully the child's wishes are consulted, will have been made by an adult. Non-directive play therapy is, we think, the least coercive of approaches because its key features, the fact that the child chooses the focus of activity and the reflective rather than interpretive stance of the therapist, means that to a considerable extent control is vested in the child rather than the therapist. Nonetheless, the therapist focuses on the child's ongoing feelings in order to bring about change in the child, and therefore by implication is attempting to influence his behaviour. Although the exercise of control is curtailed by the non-directive approach, the unequal power relationship between adult therapist and child client cannot wholly be eradicated.

In Delroy's case, there were particular features of his background and situation which made it essential to keep these issues to the fore. Not only did he suffer from a physical illness which experience and reports suggest would be likely to have exposed him to bullying and possible ridicule at school, but also, as one of the few children in the neighbourhood from a partly Afro-Caribbean background, it was likely that he would have encountered some form of racist behaviour at some time in his life. Thus it seemed important to be sensitive to issues which might have arisen from Delroy's experience of having been belittled because of his epilepsy, colour and his race. It seemed possible also that these background experiences might have left him with problems of control – either an over-readiness to please adults, which can arise when someone has learnt not to place much value on their own wishes or beliefs, or, by contrast, a stubbornness and wish to be in charge, which can occur when the child has never been allowed to feel in control.

Setting appropriate limits on his behaviour while at the same time acknowledging his right to feel and think in an individual way was, as we have seen, one of the key themes in Delroy's play therapy. One of the issues for the therapist certainly involved making sure that, in an effort not to replicate oppressive behaviour, she did not go too far in the other direction, and accede to Delroy's wishes, for example, to ignore directions as he went up to the playroom, because of anxieties about being too controlling and being experienced as oppressive.

Delroy's understanding of and problems with his racial identity, then, were hypothesised by the therapist as a potentially important theme. In their sessions, however, the therapist did not detect any direct reference to this issue. Especially when Delroy played with the black, brown and white horses in his sessions, the therapist was alert to possible 'black–white' issues and Delroy's possible identification with a particularly coloured horse. However, attachment, sexual abuse and epilepsy seemed to be the important themes of these play enactments for Delroy, not his racial identity. The therapist in passing referred to the 'white' horse and 'different coloured horses', but Delroy himself did not seem interested; therefore the therapist did not take up the issue herself.

In reviewing their sessions later, the therapist examined why an issue which seemed relevant to her at referral was not evident in her work with Delroy. Different possibilities, some more likely than others, were explored by her. Did Delroy feel inhibited in thinking about this issue because of the therapist's own Caucasian identity? – while a possibility, the therapist had worked with other mixed race children who had worked through feelings of inferiority and of rejection by themselves and others of their African ancestry as well as ways to cope with peer prejudice – or was Delroy developmentally delayed to the extent that colours were not identified easily by him? This possibility also became less likely in her opinion when Delroy readily and spontaneously identified paint colours. Did Delroy have a lack of experience and information on his racial identity? Given Jane's information about his mother's avoidance of the topic of Delroy's father, this explanation seemed a likely one and the therapist made a mental note to refer to Delroy's need for life-story work, with specific work directed to his racial identity, once his medical assessment was completed and he had settled into a more stable placement. Finally, was Delroy preoccupied with other more urgent emotional issues, also identified at referral by the therapist, which prevented him from examining his racial identity? This seemed the most likely explanation to the therapist, with Delroy's current sense of 'differentness' and negative evaluation of himself linked most directly to his epilepsy, attachment inadequacies and sexual abuse, rather than to his racial identity.

The therapist, then, has to be vigilant in allowing her hypotheses and opinions to inform her practice but, as with Delroy, not to impose them without direct evidence on the child himself. Indeed, given the severity and multiplicity of his problems, Delroy would perhaps have become even more confused if the therapist had attempted to direct his attention towards his racial identity as well.

Other personal issues for the therapist

An issue we have discussed in this book and elsewhere in different contexts (Wilson et al., 1992; Ryan and Wilson, 1995a, 1995b) is that the therapist's professional relationship with a child in non-directive play therapy is necessarily a personalised one. This method of play therapy is based on a highly empathic attitude and a deliberate intensifying of adult–child interactions.

However, in some cases, where the therapist has overstepped her professional role, as arguably the therapist had with Delroy, she may have much greater difficulty in refraining from overpersonalising her already close relationship with the child.

Several different inappropriate responses may arise, which the therapist will need help with in her supervision, as well as learning to recognise and control in her ongoing therapeutic work. One primary difficulty may be that the therapist overly stresses her own ability to help or 'rescue' the child.

Another problem for the therapist may be that in especially difficult cases other professionals can also hold their own 'rescue' fantasies. In Delroy's case it is quite possible that the foster carers and the social worker also vacilated between overcommitment to Delroy, and guilt and frustration over their inability to meet his needs. However, because these difficulties were not recognised and addressed directly, it seemed to lead to each professional becoming frustrated with the other's actions and responses, and a lack of coordinated help for Delroy. The therapist, for example, was unable to achieve even her limited goals for Delroy. This was in a small way due to his insecurity concerning transport arrangements and the lack of involvement of his foster carers in his sessions, which was, in turn, part of the wider issue of his deep need for attachments.

An added dimension in professionals' responses to Delroy's particular case is that it was readily apparent that they were working with a child with deep and multiple emotional problems, as well as a life-threatening physical condition. In addition to these factors, viable alternatives to his current short-term placement seemed non-existent. Many avenues of help had been explored by his social worker and her managers, yet the necessary resources for Delroy in their locale simply were not found. The therapist did seem mistaken, in retrospect, for not concentrating on offering consultations with the professionals already involved in Delroy's life and helping them towards a more cohesive approach to his care. It was doubtful, however, that this offer would have been taken up, because of both carers' and social services' perceptions of Delroy's needs. Because of her decision to begin work, and then her decision not to renegotiate her role with the social worker and carers, partly because of the short-term nature of her intervention, the therapist was left in the very dubious position of intervening and attempting to shore up an unviable foster placement for a child. Even in retrospect, however, it is very difficult to see a clear, effective plan of action for Delroy by the therapist that would have been more likely to have been productive.

In some cases, regretfully, no answers are forthcoming and the therapist – as the social worker and foster carers – tries to work within her abilities, at what she is allowed to do, and under conditions which are not favourable ones to begin with (Ryan, 1995b). The reader will have to make his or her own personal judgement in Delroy's case, and perhaps have the advantage of greater distance from the issues, and greater experience or expertise than the authors, in arriving at strategies for a more workable intervention.

Chapter 6

Patricia

Reworking Abusive Experiences in Adolescence

*To know this, and know that however ugly the parts appear
The whole remains beautiful. A severed hand
Is an ugly thing...*

Robinson Jeffers 'Not man apart'

FIRST ENCOUNTERS

Patricia entered the playroom with assurance, sat down readily on the upholstered easy chair, removed her coat and folded it neatly, then carefully crossed her legs at the knee and glanced up at me, as if signalling that I should begin. She looked older that her 13 years, physically mature, with fair hair carefully fluffed up round her face, pale lipstick and violet eyeshadow. As I started talking, she studiedly ignored me, examining her well-manicured and polished finger nails, then pushing down the cuticles rhythmically on each hand. I limited myself to brief remarks, reminding her that when I had met her I'd said that she would be able to use her time with me as she wanted, and that I'd also talked about needing to tell social services if children and young people I worked with told me about the dangerous or damaging things that happened to them. She scanned the room and returned to me.

P: Well, it gets me a ride home from school at any rate.
V: You're not sure this is a good idea but you'll try it out.

Patricia nodded, saying it was much too far to walk to her foster home from school anyway, and she should be getting a lift every day. I reflected her feeling that she didn't feel very well taken care of as far as that was concerned, and that maybe some things in her life now seemed difficult.

These first reflections of her feelings were made easier for me and I felt

I was finding the right things to say to her, partly because of the information which Matthew, her social worker, had earlier discussed with me. At our referral meeting, he had told me that Patricia would not be at all intimidated by me and that she was more than able to say what she thought. However, there were signs that, in spite of her articulate and self-confident manner, she was troubled and less sure of herself than she appeared. She would benefit from some time with a professional separate from social services to help her come to terms with her admission into care.

Matthew confided that he found Patricia's family particularly difficult to work with constructively. He felt himself pushed in his relationship with the family and with Patricia into being an authoritarian figure who enforces rules. Everyone in the family argued and criticised one another, but with him around they became united in a concerted attempt to undermine his authority in every conceivable way possible. Patricia was already expert at this, and seemed to have been taught by her family that animosity towards professionals and towards social workers in particular, was both a requirement if you were to be counted as a member of the family and essential for the family's survival. This attitude pervaded her extended family as well and could in part be explained by the fact that social services had for some time been suspicious that Patricia's cousins were being sexually abused by several of her adult relatives. A number of investigations had been carried out and were recorded on file, but none of them had proved conclusive. Matthew said that the atmosphere in several of these related families seemed to be highly charged, with sexual inuendoes and very explicit sexual language from both adults and children. There was a total lack of disciplining of the children's behaviour or language by the adult members of the family.

They were also a very close knit family in adversity. The extended family had been outraged when the mother of a close friend of Patricia's had decided to inform social services of what Patricia had told her daughter had been happening to her. Patricia had confided to her friend that her uncle had sexually abused her when she was younger and now she was being abused by her step-father. She had needed to talk about her experiences because she was afraid that her uncle was beginning to show signs of intending to abuse her six-year-old half brother, Shaun, who had a mild learning disability. Patricia had said to her friend that she was worried about Shaun because her family operated that way – it had happened to her mother when she was a child, then it had been her 16-year-old sister's turn, and then hers. Soon she would be too old and it would be Shaun. However, Patricia had refused to discuss anything with the original social worker doing the investigation and, when she had been received into care, her family had made threats on the social worker's life.

This social worker had therefore been removed from Patricia's case and Matthew had taken it over.

Matthew also discussed with me his frustration over current child protection issues in Patricia's family. Although there had been enough evidence for the judge to decide that Patricia needed an Emergency Protection Order, she had refused to repeat or confirm her allegations during the joint investigative interview with the previous social worker and a police officer. So although the courts had made an interim Care Order on Patricia, no criminal proceedings were viable, and Shaun remained at home on a Supervision Order. Matthew continued to worry that, predictably, Patricia's mother did not seem to be protecting Shaun adequately from his father or uncle, even though she had agreed that her brother, Shaun's uncle, would not have any contact with him and that she would not leave Shaun alone in his father's company. (Matthew concurred when I expressed concern at the potential risks to Shaun in leaving him at home, given that his father remained there too.) Until there was more proof available, or until family assessments had been done and a final hearing for care orders on Patricia and Shaun had been heard, this very unsatisfactory situation would continue. Patricia was in a foster home, but resented having been placed in care, saying it was not fair that Shaun should remain at home and she had had to leave. Although Matthew had talked to her about this and the other issues involved, which included Patricia's own failure to accept her mother's authority over her at home and wanting to have all the privileges of her 16-year-old sister, she remained very angry with him personally. Perhaps a woman counsellor who had no statutory role would be able to work more productively with her.

I was interested in helping Patricia, and since her foster placement was potentially a long-term one where she would stay until she was 18, it gave her the necessary stability to examine her feelings. I collected written background reports from Matthew, including the assessment report by a child and adolescent psychiatrist written after he had interviewed Patricia, and arranged to meet Patricia herself, her mother and foster carers before our sessions began.

PATRICIA'S PLAY THERAPY SESSIONS

Patricia's initial sessions, as even the first few minutes with her described above highlight, were marked by her unusual poise and use of very direct language. During her 15 sessions she returned repeatedly to several themes that were emotionally important to her. Sometimes these issues were readily detected within the sessions as single concerns, and at other times they merged together and would then diverge again.

Patricia's changing attitudes towards the therapist, and the testing out of her trustworthiness and consistency as an adult was one key concern thoughout her sessions. Another theme which emerged during her therapy was her use of play therapy materials to work through her abusive experiences on an immediate, bodily level; this seemed also to awaken her deeper childhood memories and sensations. Related to this theme was a third theme involving Patricia's development of relationships with her foster carers which were emotionally very different from those with adult members of her own family. (The first two themes have been discussed briefly in Ryan, 1995a.)

After discussing Patricia's sessions in terms of these themes, we shall draw practice concerns from her story. Our primary focus will be the ways in which play therapy can be sensitive to the needs of adolescent clients. The final section on theoretical issues will discuss adolescent emotional needs and their relationship to play therapy, and will explore our theoretical understanding of the way in which play therapy alters mental structures by working on motor levels as well as on cognitive and affective ones.

Confidentiality and the development of trust

Patricia began her sessions by putting herself firmly in control. She readily engaged in conversation with me, and seemed to thrive in an atmosphere in which she was the one who directed the conversation and activities rather than the adult. She also seemed to enjoy my attention as I reflected her ongoing feelings back to her. Taking the lead in our early conversations, she freely expressed her negative feelings towards social services. She ridiculed Matthew, thinking up one insulting caricature after another to describe his appearance and manner, while I listened (with an internal smile of admiration for her skill at mimicry) and reflected her strong feelings of anger and contempt for him. Patricia went on to blame both her friend's mother and social services for the 'terrible' interview she'd been subjected to with the social workers and police, saying several times, 'As if I'd tell them *anything* about my family'. She also compared the actions of these professionals to her family's, saying what they'd done to her had been far worse than anything she'd had done to her in her family. She went on to berate social services for removing her from home, saying her mum and Johnny (her step-dad) said it didn't make any sense to remove her and leave Shaun at home. As she expressed her feelings, she continually asked me what I felt about it, did I think it was fair, didn't I think she should be at home . . . I tried to answer her questions as honestly and as briefly as I could, while still giving precedence to Patricia's own thoughts and feelings. For example:

> P: None of you know how it feels when your Mum's not there.
> V: It isn't happening to *us*. *You're* the one who's hurting inside from it all.
> P: You don't think somebody my age should have to get on all alone, do you?
> V: No. You have Sarah and Michael looking after you, but you feel you need your Mum, not them. You're very lonely in your foster home without your Mum.

Often, however, her questions to me seemed rhetorical, or she would listen and then engage in another assault on professionals if she heard me presenting a view not in agreement with her own. She repeated often that I couldn't possibly know her or what she felt, and how difficult it was for her in foster care. And that I didn't know and love her family and miss them like she did. I persisted in agreeing with her that she had her own understandings and feelings, that I was trying to understand and share with her what I thought when she wanted me to, and that she felt very hurt by all that had happened.

As well as this verbal barrage and quizzing, Patricia by her second session began to scrutinise my face intently when she paused to think. Because at these times Patricia waited until I glanced down or away, I sensed that she did not want me to meet her gaze. I therefore remained still, making my face available for her to examine, but feeling a bit stripped of my skin. I used this feeling to reflect back what seemed to be her own feeling of wanting to get right inside me and know me, and of feeling puzzled by me.

> P: When I went to see the 'nut doctor', you know that one that locks people up in the nut house, he just wanted to hear all about the sex thing.
> V: You're worried that I might be like him. Even though I've said this is time for you to use the way you want, you think I might really just want to know about the sexual abuse, like he did.
> P: That's all he was on about, and what the police and all of them social workers are always on about, too.
> V: Maybe it's not important for you to talk about the 'sex thing' with me. But if it is some time, I'll listen and try and help you with your feelings if you want me to. But it's up to you, what you say here.

Patricia became uncharacteristically quiet for a time, and manipulating the clay ball that she had had in her hand from the start, began to knead and squeeze it while we talked. Matching her thoughtful mood, I paused too, saying to her quietly after a time that she seemed to be sorting out what she thought about what we'd said.

As our sessions progressed, Patricia began to expand on her feelings towards social services. Having given vent to her anger, and mistrust of professionals and of social workers in particular, she began to put to one side the attitudes which she had adopted from her family and become more personal. She still felt that it was very unfair for social services to have removed her from home, but she began to wonder why social services believed the information she had given to the psychiatrist, saying that her family, and especially Johnny and her uncle, were so believable that *anybody* would take their word over hers. She hadn't told the nut doctor too much, but she'd said they had made her touch them. I helped her to realise that these two ideas were difficult to put together for her – why would social services believe her and yet her family wouldn't accept what she said?

Struggling with her strong emotions, Patricia said in a strangulated voice that her family had said they didn't want her back until she 'told the truth'. I said that Patricia was desperate to go home, but her family were making her lie to be with them again. Patricia began weeping, then turned angrily to me and said with venom, through her tears, that I'd just let her cry and not do anything about it. 'You're useless!' she shouted at me. 'You can't understand what I feel or you'd *do* something about it!' After her outburst, I talked to her in a warm but gentle voice, saying how painful it was to see how much she was suffering and that I would like to make it all right for her, but that I couldn't change her family for her. Only her family could do that for themselves.

Patricia continued to show she was angry with me throughout the rest of the session, but stopped crying. She told me several times in different contexts that I was useless, and I reflected that she was angry with me, that in her opinion I couldn't do things very well, that I wasn't being what she wanted me to be for her. By the end of the session, the intensity of these statements had diminished but not stopped. She left at the end of the session criticising the way I always got up to leave, mimicking my manner and accent, saying, 'Don't say it, I will. "Well, I guess we have to go downstairs now, Patricia"', in mocking tones. I replied, 'That hurts my feelings just a bit, if you make fun of me'.

During our next few sessions, Patricia returned to the same topic, gradually becoming much less angry with me as she tentatively began to admit to herself that her family wasn't very honest with her about a lot of things – she couldn't trust what her mum said to her about her step-dad, that her aunty and her gran said different things about her uncle from those Johnny and her grandad said. She talked about a cousin of hers who had gone away last year, who wasn't much older than she was, and how she'd had different stories from all the adults about it; it was only her other cousin who'd told her the truth, that he'd been put in care because he'd been hit. Patricia also began to wonder whether the information she'd received from her mother and Johnny about what social workers had said to them was true. I again tried to help her with these feelings, recognising her frustration with me for not providing her with answers to her questions about her family and reflecting her anxiety that she had no older members of her family that she felt able to turn to for the truth.

Although she used me as an anchor while she explored her conflicting emotions and confused thoughts about herself and her relationship with her family, she was still very mistrustful of my professional role. Along with family issues, she continually brought up, often in a verbally hostile way, many of her concerns about the confidentiality of our sessions together. She needed to hear from me repeatedly that I used my audio-recordings of the sessions to write out notes and that I then erased the tapes. I also explained on several different occasions that these sessional notes were for my own use to remember our time together and that no one else would see them. I told her the exceptions to this rule would be if a judge ordered me to turn my notes over to the court or if I was asked in court about my time with her. I had also told her at the beginning, that if she herself told me something that involved serious hurt to her or other people I would have to tell social services. We also discussed several times in our early sessions the reports I would write for social services and I repeated each time that I would write a general report for her social services file after ten sessions together, when I knew her better. In this I would say what progress she was making, whether I was helping her, what general things concerned her and what she needed in the short- and long-term future. I illustrated each point with an example, talked about how maybe Patricia didn't trust adults because she didn't know the truth and they kept secrets from her. Because it was so important to her that she had accurate information from me, and because of her age and understanding, I offered to go through any report or information with her beforehand that I planned to share with social services or the court. We could talk about what I was planning to say and she could give me her opinion about it.

Patricia did not accept my assurances easily. She often challenged me during our sessions about whether I was going to tell Matthew about her behaviour or what she had said, being especially concerned as to whether I would share with him the contempt she felt for him (half hoping I would!) She was most anxious that I didn't share with him her doubts and negative feelings about her family, or her anger towards me. It was only towards the end of our first group of ten sessions (we had 15 rather than 20 for reasons discussed later) that she said to me in a somewhat defiant manner, which seemed apprehensive underneath, that she'd had lots of secrets from me during our sessions. She said, with a mixture of triumph and uncertainty, that she'd kept to herself some of the 'chicken' games she'd started playing with her new friends in the neighbourhood, like running over railway tracks when the signals had gone red. They'd stopped now: it was just for a while. She admitted liking having secrets from me, and besides, she knew if she'd told me I'd have gone straight to Matthew and told on her.

I smiled and said that now she knew me better and could tell me, that it had been fun then to know she was more powerful than me; maybe she felt I was like a lot of other adults then, trying to find out too much about her and she needed to have some important secrets from me. Patricia nodded thoughtfully. I added that Patricia had been right to take me at my word. That I did think my job as an adult was to help teenagers, and part of that would be to try to stop them doing things that would harm themselves or others. I probably would have had to tell someone else, if I had thought what she was doing was really dangerous.

She also approached her concern about confidentiality tangentially in most of our first ten sessions, using her interest in other children's activities with me in the playroom to test out my resolve about keeping to my rule that what happened in the sessions was private. This rule and my adherence to it seemed to be a continuing irritant to Patricia, and emotionally very important to her. I talked to her about how her curiosity was aroused, her sense of powerlessness keenly felt, and her belief that if she persisted, my resolve would be weakened. I began inwardly to feel harrassed by her. She was certainly skillful in her tactics, probably imitating ploys which adults had used towards her in close relationships, and showing the practice she already had herself in this kind of erosion of another's resolve. As well as feeling badgered by Patricia, I was also intrigued to see that her feelings and thoughts were very fluid around this issue. She seemed to use such a variety of logical arguments – that it wouldn't matter very much to another child if she knew about the child playing in the sand, that she wouldn't tell anyone else, that other children might like her interest in them – and such a variety of feelings – genuine interest in others, frustration with me, powerlessness, determination and a sense of purpose. Her tactics changed from persuasive, more abstract arguments to a young child's appealing, wheedling tone. I felt my own skill and sense of purpose thoroughly taxed by her, as I tried to give her my reasons clearly, without becoming unduly weighed down by logical arguments and verbage. Above all, I tried to help Patricia understand her own emotions which were so varied, and made the issue so important to her. These included her changing feelings towards my responses and my adult authority and the need to protect children's privacy in my relationships with them. For example, in one session she commented that the playdough had been mixed together again, and asked:

P: Did that girl I see downstairs sometimes, did she use it?
V: You're still very curious about what other children do here. Even though I've told you lots of times that I try to keep other children's time

with me private, just like yours, you still want to know.
P: But did she? It won't matter just telling me that.
V: I try to keep my word with children when I say this is private time. I think that's very important. But you keep coming back to it, feeling frustrated with me when I don't tell you about anyone else. And you don't see why I should be in charge and make the rule.

Towards the end of our first ten sessions, Patricia seemed to have accepted my stand on privacy for others and by implication herself, and had a somewhat begrudging trust in me, as evidenced by her telling me about the dangerous games she had been playing. She then shifted towards a greater degree of emotional openness and genuine trust, telling me about how glad she'd been when she came that I was a woman. It had been so difficult to talk with the male psychiatrist during her assessment, and her bad luck, she still had Matthew, 'that pain in the arse'. She wanted to talk some more to me about what had really 'gotten to her' the most and made her tell her friend. She said some of it she'd thought was fun, even though it was scary, but when her step-dad had kept insisting she push at him and the yuck would come out, she would feel sort of sick and disgusted about it all and want to just wash and wash her hands, over and over again. She still wished she hadn't left home – she did miss her mum and Shaun so much, and she was so lonely for her own bed and her own things in her room. 'Besides, everybody at home says they know it's my fault Johnny and Steve [her uncle] can't do lots of things at home any more. So no-one feels sorry at all for me. They think it serves me right to be in care.'

Patricia's reworking of sexually abusive experiences on a bodily level

However, to describe our sessions as only discussions between Patricia and me would be misleading. She developed her trust and openness verbally, but it seemed equally important to her to be able to make use of the play materials in the room and in doing so to resolve some of her emotional conflicts on a bodily level. In our early sessions, as we talked, Patricia's hands often worked independently and unconsciously, busily manipulating clay, softening it, squeezing it, relaxing it and releasing it. Sometimes our conversation would come to a pause and she would centre her attention on the consistency of the formless shape in her hands, add water to make it smooth, and work the clay into a simple shape — a ball, a slope, an arch — stroking the sleek, wet curves. Then she would begin to look at them closely and critically, saying how babyish and 'useless' they were. As I reflected her dissatisfaction with what her hands could do, Patricia would begin another conversation with me, squeezing her clay shapeless again in her hands.

After a few sessions which were dominated by her talk, she began to shift her attention more often towards her hands' activities. She began to smooth the wet clay over both her hands, covering them completely and remaining silent, concentrating, as I quietly commented to her on the way the clay felt and the way her hands felt, too, completely covered up, hidden and different inside. She would then wait, allowing the clay covering to harden completely, then making it crack and flake as she wriggled her fingers.

> V: Making it break up; your fingers want to be free of it. They seem trapped inside. [Patricia grimaced, looking down at her hands as she moved them.]
> V: Not liking it now.

Silently, Patricia would go to the basin in the room, remove her watch and scrub her hands and finger nails repeatedly.

> V: It's so difficult to get them clean, the way you want them, when they've become so covered up and hardened. You have to make such a big effort.

I thought to myself, with my own thoughts as sober as Patricia's seemed to be: perhaps what I had observed from our beginning session, that Patricia's hands seemed unconnected to her mind and yet very busy with their own activities, was now being made more visible, and becoming more connected for her. The symbolic link to her sexual abuse, being relived through her hands, in my presence, seemed strong. It seemed important for her that we both remained silent, not voicing our thoughts. As she continued her coating and cleansing activities, repeating them in each session, and as I continued to reflect the same emotive messages to her, she began to give me small tasks to help her with – holding her watch, rolling up her sleeves, getting another paper towel. I sensed I was being more accepted, in my helping role, as long as she felt in control of how I helped. I began to reflect this to her gradually.

> P: [Hands dripping] Get me another one, will you.
> V: [Handing her a paper towel] You're letting me help, instead of just standing by while you do all the work.
> P: I'm not one of those little ones you see, you know.
> V: You're in charge. You're old enough to do it all, but sometimes you let me help to make it easier for you. [Inadvertently, Patricia smiled a secret smile of shy pleasure at my getting it right.]

Patricia soon branched out to other materials, first using playdough and remembering happy times in her childhood with playdough, feeling close to her mother and close to everyone in her family. As I spoke to her, matching my light tone to hers, she began to get angry, once more verbally attacking the social worker for removing her from home.

V: You're wishing it were still that way; and feeling angry with the social worker because you want to be happy at home and want so much that your mum and everyone in your family love you.

Next, she substituted finger paints for clay, using the same technique, but this time layering her hands with one bright colour after another, until her hands became coated again, with the colours merging into a sticky turgid brown sludge. In the process of coating her hands with the bright colours, Patricia's body moved in a swaying, sensual motion and I said how good the stroking, smooth paint felt to her; she was enjoying it so much that her body felt good all over. As the paint thickened and the colours changed, I talked about how Patricia kept going on, losing the nice colours she'd enjoyed at the beginning, but didn't seem able to stop. Then I reflected her disgust with her sticky, messy, muddy-looking hands when she finished, and how she quickly had to scrub until all the paint was gone and her hands looked pretty and clean again. I always spoke briefly, using few words, almost to myself, but with feeling.

As Patricia returned to her ritualised hand painting in her next sessions, she began to relax somewhat, her hand motions becoming less frantic and less prolonged. She was uncharacteristically silent, yet her movements continued without self-consciousness or restraint. The only mention she made herself directly to me about these hand-painting sequences was to ensure as she left each week that I would replenish the finger paints for her next time. I assured her that I knew the paints were very important to her and that I'd make sure she had some for as long as she needed them. Patricia used the paints for several sessions before returning to modelling with clay, this time modelling small animal statues for her friends at school. I was interested to note to myself, for Patricia didn't refer to it herself, that her appearance was changing from that of a meticulously groomed, poised and self-contained young adult into a young teenager experimenting with casual hair and casual dress which was much more similar to other 13-year-old girls.

Relationships with peers and other significant adults

Although not calling attention in her sessions to her changing appearance, Patricia did mention her school friends frequently. She talked about how supportive other girls in her class were to her, feeling grateful for their support and comfort when she had to leave home. Patricia had been concerned at her first session that she might get teased by them for attending therapy sessions; I had acknowledged this anxiety with her and we discussed practical strategies for minimising their knowledge of her sessions, including timing our sessions for her lunch hour; she would think it over. Patricia returned triumphantly for her second session, announcing that everyone was envying her for going out during school time and doing art work.

Her discussions about boys of her own age were much more conflicting than those about girls. She repeatedly and vehemently denied any sexual interest in adolescent boys she knew, without my having said anything at all about them. Yet she returned often to describing, with obvious feelings of satisfaction and even triumph, incidents in which she had deliberately encouraged these boys to make sexual advances towards her and then aggressively rejected and ridiculed them. As she described these incidents in a dramatic manner, I made tentative attempts briefly to reflect some of her feelings, talking about her wanting the boys to think she was attractive and that they would like to have her as a girlfriend, but hating them when they made passes, or tried to pull at her blouse. But she soon made it very clear that my comments were not acceptable. My role was to listen and, she hoped, to provide an appreciative audience. While Patricia could discuss these encounters without embarrassment, she remained unable to tolerate any comments from me about her strong, conflicting sexual feelings. She seemed to want to avoid thinking about her feelings and motives; instead she wanted me to think her first daring, and then justified, in her responses. I said that I couldn't give her praise and admiration, as I felt she wanted from me, but that I could understand how she was feeling. Patricia became angry with me, saying I hadn't been there and couldn't ever know what she was feeling about anything. I said, 'I know for certain that you're angry with me now!' She tossed her head, then looked back at me more thoughtfully and did not return to her exploits again.

Another time when Patricia became angry with me was when my own feelings about her foster carer, Michael, differed from her own. Patricia accepted my reflections easily at the beginning about Michael, about her newly forming affectionate feeling for him, and her gratitude and amazement that he would comfort her when sadness about being separated from her mother and family overwhelmed her. She began to contrast him with her step-dad, Johnny, and other men in her extended family, including her uncle. She began to acknowledge to herself that she felt superior to Johnny because she was free of him now but she was sure that he still thought he needed her; but jealous of him too, because her mum seemed to be loving him more than her and putting him first.

She began to talk about the men in her family being weak and helpless underneath, even though they threatened and blustered all the time. Michael didn't do any of those things, but she thought he was genuinely strong and she could count on him. Patricia's anger with me came out at this point. After the session, she and I always walked out to where

Michael and his wife Sarah were waiting in their car for her and she knew that I had gone to a meeting with Michael, Sarah and Matthew recently. (One of the issues which we had all discussed at this meeting had been Michael's concerns over Patricia's deepening feelings towards him, and how he and Sarah could help her maintain a normal, asexual and affectionate relationship with an adult male carer, which she was seeking and so much needed to replace the abusive relationships she had developed with adult men in her family.)

Patricia urged me to say that I thought Michael was kind and loving, and wanted me to send him a birthday card as she was planning to do. I replied that I knew she felt that way about him and he was special to her, but I didn't have that kind of relationship with him. Patricia started berating me, telling me that I knew her and should feel like she did. I answered that I'd like to agree with her about my feelings because it was so important to her, but that I couldn't change the way I felt about it or lie about it. She listened intently, perhaps thinking of the demands her own family made on her to conform to their attitudes towards other adult family members who were abusing her, although she didn't verbalise any of her thoughts to me so that I could be more certain. She did, though, begin to realise and accept that I would be able to tolerate – as would Sarah – her affection for Michael without having identical relationships ourselves with him. And she could begin to acknowledge to herself that Michael, and Sarah, too, were becoming important to her.

The Easter holidays were coming soon and we talked about one more session before the holidays, taking a break for two weeks, then resuming the five sessions for which we still had funding after that. Patricia said in a very matter-of-fact tone, which seemed to signal that she had already made her decision, that she'd come for the last time next week. I told her I thought there were a few problems (thinking about her relations with adolescent boys in particular) which she might still find me useful to help her with still, but she forestalled any discussion of issues, saying she missed being at school and wanted to be part of things. She'd had enough now. I said I wanted to do what seemed best for her: I would talk with Matthew, Michael and Sarah about what she'd said, and we could talk about it again next week. She could also have that time to think some more if she needed it. Patricia's decision didn't alter during the week, and in my talk with her carers and social worker, we had all agreed that she was continuing to make progress, and that barring unforseen events this was likely to go on. We parted with a hug, exhuberantly initiated by Patricia.

Two years later, I happened to meet Patricia's new social worker, who had been working with her for the past year. She told me that, despite some setbacks in foster care and some current difficulties with boyfriends, she had continued to make real progress. She seemed able to turn to her carers when she needed to talk things over, had developed in confidence and maturity at school, and to my great delight, her social worker was optimistic that her progress would continue.

PRACTICE ISSUES

Adapting play therapy to the needs of adolescents

Play therapy has traditionally been regarded as an approach to be used with children, and there are few accounts of the way in which it can be adapted and used as an effective intervention with young adolescents. We hope that Patricia's story will provide just such an illustration, and in this section, we want to consider the kinds of adaptations which the therapist usually needs to make in working with adolescents and with some older children.

Non-directive play therapy has its roots in Rogerian, client-centred counselling, as we, among others, have shown. In our earlier book, we said that it is based on many of the same principles of development and understanding of the way in which therapeutic change occurs as Rogerian counselling, but that in it play rather than speech is the principal medium of communication. We also tried to develop a theoretical means of understanding how it is that play therapy works, and how play itself fits into this theoretical framework, pointing out that, in child developmental terms, play is a highly adaptive activity, and one of the main ways in which children develop understandings and explore conflicts. This use of symbolic play as an assimilative activity gradually diminishes during adolescence, as the capacity for verbalisation and inner thought becomes established. By adulthood, this kind of play has largely disappeared. Clearly adults do use play to meet a variety of goals, from kinetic to social exchange purposes. However, with, among other changes during adolescence, the acquisition of more complex and abstract mental abilities, symbolic play as a general adaptive activity largely ceases. Instead, verbal exchanges and inner thought largely take its place, and it seems likely in adult counselling that verbal metaphor and images, often used by the therapist in response to the client's communications, take on this transforming role and function.

It is for this reason that therapeutic approaches with adolescents have largely focused on counselling or other more adult-oriented therapies rather than play therapy. However, for reasons based both on our practice and on our theoretical understanding, an approach which encompasses both action and talk seems well adapted to addressing adolescent problems. Indeed, the practice of art and drama therapies suggests that approaches which allow for creative and motor responses, in the way that play therapy does, have their usefulness with adults, too.

We acknowledge, however, that the term 'play' may be off-putting to adolescents. Perhaps a term such as 'creative' or 'personal' therapy would be more acceptable, and respect their sensitivity to others' recognition of their more mature status, which we discuss below.

There are good reasons, then, for using a play therapy approach in working with adolescents, based on a developmental perspective of adolescence as being the midway point between childhood and adulthood. Young people who have experienced childhood traumas, stresses or discontinuities also have particular developmental needs which make play therapy appropriate. It is important, however, for the therapist to anticipate, in preparing for the work and in undertaking it, certain concerns which may arise for this age group. Because adolescents are often uncertain of their social status, no longer regarding themselves as children but not yet having acquired adult roles, or in early adolescence even some of the social confidence of middle and late adolescence, adolescents can be especially sensitive to situations which attempt to treat them as children. On the other hand, a room which is wholly geared for adults may easily be dismissed as 'boring'. In any case the therapist still needs, as with younger children, to select activities which lend themselves to unstructured symbolic activities and play.

As we said in our earlier book, it is important therefore to ensure that the adolescents feel their age is being respected, while at the same time engendering the same sense of permissiveness needed with a younger child. So it is worth thinking about the initial impact of the room – does it look so geared to small children that the teenager will feel s/he really doesn't belong here? Is the furniture adult sized, preferably with some comfortable easy chairs, and at least a few structured activities for an older age group (jigsaws, board games) so that the adolescent doesn't feel demeaned by what is on offer? As with younger age groups, materials (such as art materials, puppets and dressing-up materials) should be selected which can be used in an advanced way as well as materials which can be used for much younger, regressive play. Some materials seem particularly well adapted for older children and early adolescence; playdough and clay can, as we saw with Patricia, be manipulated and modelled while talking; soft balls can be kicked around or used in organised games; playing cards can be used for magic tricks or card games with the therapist; puppets can be used to stage plays; and paints, chalks and other drawing materials can be used for symbolic representations.

The room therefore, needs to be organised in a way that shows that it can be used by children and young people of different ages both to sit and talk, and also to play in. Provided that the sessions are conducted in a way which is sensitive to the adolescents' need not to be treated as children, but with a permissiveness which allows them to feel free either to talk, or to play with what is available if they wish to do so, then it is usually possible to assuage any initial reservations, and to engage them therapeutically, despite their worries about looking 'babyish' to outsiders.

As we discuss in the next theoretical section on the development of identity in adolescence, an important feature of this process is the integration of past experiences into an emerging sense of adult identity. An adolescent may feel cut off and prohibited from using children's toys, games and behaviour, and yet may still need, even if only fleetingly, to return to the earlier experiences represented by them. Many adolescent children will engage in vigorous physical games with their younger siblings while at the same time declaring their total boredom and impatience with this and later returning to more grown-up pursuits. However, for adolescents whose earlier relationships have in some ways been damaging, the need to get in touch with and to rework earlier stages of development, is often critical. A particular advantage of non-directive play therapy is that the way in which the sessions are conducted easily allows for this reintegration of past experiences into current life and experiences. By having available materials suitable for children of different ages, the adolescent is more easily reminded of different stages in his or her own development. For this reason, it is important to include in the playroom materials which will allow this to occur if the teenager chooses, such as dolls and a doll's house, tea set, baby's bottle, bricks, farm animals, small figures and so on. Within the sessions, then, adolescents can suck the baby's bottle, play with dolls in the doll's house, organise mock battles with guns, use finger paints and dress up, much as younger children do when they relive their past experiences or fantasies. Other adolescents and older children may choose to use the materials, on the other hand, in more socially acceptable ways – the dressing up clothes being used for 'plays' or charades, and the doll's house being set up 'for the children who come' and not for themselves to play with. Unlike other more directive methods, or those based more exclusively on verbal or cognitive approaches, the adolescents can choose materials and activites appropriate to themselves, and the appropriate time for their use, without outside pressure or the fear of losing face.

Patricia in fact seemed to have no difficulty in accepting the play setting or materials as appropriate for her age. Given her very poised and mature appearance, this seemed to the therapist in itself noteworthy. She hypothesised that this contrast between Patricia's outward appearance and her readiness to use play materials might reflect a greater hesitation and uncertainty about the mature self which she presented to the world, and that she might in fact feel less assured and grown up than she appeared. Her initial worries centred instead, as we have seen, on her own use of the materials, which she felt to be clumsy and rather babyish, and anxieties about being teased by her school friends for needing therapy at all.

We have seen in the other case studies how many of these children focus on one medium of play for a time, and then move into another type of activity, often one which is in some way more personal to them. Thus Diane's play in her early sessions mainly involved painting the balloon, and she only fleetingly dressed up, using situations to enact which were to begin with only marginally personal to her, only later moving to invent more intimate sequences. Adolescents' use of play materials often seems to follow a similar progression, with early activities focusing at a more impersonal or more cognitive level, and later changing to activities which seem to represent more intense and intimate issues for them. One 14 year old, for example, whose sessions started mostly on a verbal level, moved to doing representational paintings and drawings, before gravitating to the doll's house, where she enacted intense sequences of play with the family of dolls.

Patricia's curiosity about the other children who used the play therapy room suggested, as well as a testing out of the therapist's reliability in observing confidentiality, some need to remember and/or re-experience for herself what it felt like to be a child. The sequence of these explorations also seems significant, in that much of her exploration was conducted first at a verbal level, with intense questioning about what these children did, and with the clay being used as an adjunct to verbal exchanges with the therapist. She seemed to concentrate on these as she moulded the clay into simple figures, and then worked them into smooth curves and squeezed them shapeless again. Only after a time did she move on to use clay and finger paints more intensively, in what seemed to be a reworking of her experiences and memories at a motor and relatively unconscious level, and during this phase her verbalisations became much less prominent. The availability of the different materials, and the acceptance by the therapist of both talking and play materials as a means of expression and exploration, allowed her to move between the different mediums as she wished and felt ready to do so.

An essential part of lessening the adolescent's inhibitions in trying out different ways of exploring their experiences is to build a sense of confidence in the privacy provided by the setting, and of trust in the therapist. We saw with Patricia that privacy and confidentiality were extremely preoccupying for her, and surmise that this partly arose because of the particular dynamics around secrets, from other family members and from the outside world, within her own family. However, even if these issues do not always have quite the same emotional saliency as they did for her, most teenagers are highly sensitive to the thought of it being known that they are having therapy at all. This can include being seen going into the therapy room, so that ensuring that the room is properly private and not overlooked does help break down early reservations. The adolescent may be worried about peers' or others' possible misuse of the information that they are seeing a therapist, by teasing or labelling them as mad or, as in Patricia's case, 'nutty'. It is helpful, usually at the introductory meeting, to think through what others can be told as a 'cover' story (and as we saw in the first chapter, this is often relevant with younger children, too). In Patricia's case, she decided to say that she was having extra art sessions. Others may find less loss of face in having extra help with some aspect of school work. Potential difficulties can be helped by arranging sessions at times which do not make absence too obvious, say at lunchtime or after school.

As with other children, the reverse side of this need for confidentiality is that adolescents who have been abused may be particularly sensitive to the suggestion that the therapy sessions are shrouded in secrecy, since too much privacy in one-to-one interactions may be reminiscent of their abusive experiences. It is important to give a clear message that, although the therapist will keep the sessions confidential, within limits, the adolescent is free to talk about what happens as he or she wishes.

As with younger children, the therapist needs to make clear the circumstances in which she will need to share information about what has been communicated in the sessions. This is a much more involved issue for children in care than for someone like Anna (chapter 4), who is living with natural parent(s) and is seen outside a statutory setting. We saw with Patricia that testing the therapist's resolve over this was a powerful theme in her sessions. With many adolescents, their concerns about what others may be told about them becomes a live issue in therapy in a way that it rarely is for younger children. They have not only the intellectual ability to consider the implications of, for example, the therapist writing about the sessions for a court report, but also in any case their particular stage of development, with all its concerns about developing an identity separate, and therefore to some extent concealed, from their families, makes confidentiality a critical issue.

We look in chapters 2 and 7 at ways in which the therapist may be able to minimise these difficulties somewhat and suggest, for example, that it may sometimes be possible to cite a less sensitive, and therefore less embarrassing, example as evidence for a general statement. However, with certain things, the therapist, in balancing the long-term interests of the adolescents against the impact on them of sharing sensitive material, may decide that information needs to be shared, even if this spoils or lessens the effectiveness of therapy. In Patricia's case, for example, the therapist felt it essential that the court be informed of her opinion that Patricia had been sexually abused and emotionally damaged by members of her family. She also reported Patricia's pain at altering some of her views about her family's behaviour, although she also described Patricia's continuing love for her mother and brother. During the sessions, a more immediate concern of Patricia's was whether or not the therapist would divulge to Matthew, her social worker, the occasions when she had cried, and had felt most conscious of seeming weak and vulnerable. In this case, the therapist felt comfortable in reassuring her: there was no need, either for child protection or for future care planning, that the details of these episodes be divulged. Instead, she explained that she would be outlining to him Patricia's sadness and conflicts over loving her family and wanting to be with them and their not believing her. (See chapter 7 for a more detailed discussion.)

The adolescent's more sophisticated understanding of confidentiality does, realistically, mean that on some occasions the limited confidentiality which the therapist can offer has a restricting effect on the therapy, and may make it a more guarded and superficial relationship than it otherwise would have been. The other side of this, however, is that the sense that an adult is concerned enough to exercise some authority, and that adults have a continuing responsibility to protect adolescents from danger can also be reassuring. We saw with Patricia that the refusal to talk about other children eventually produced a rather grudging trust in what the therapist said. She also was impressed by the fact that adults had been prepared to take note of and act on what she had said about her family. With other adolescents the fact that adults are ready to act and take responsibility for their actions can come as a relief, even if it then leaves them free to blame the adults for whatever outcome occurs.

Testing the therapist's resolve over respecting the privacy of others was thus an important component of a key theme for Patricia throughout her sessions, namely establishing whether or not the therapist was a trustworthy and reliable adult. Another aspect of this is that the therapist needs to be sufficiently accurate in reflecting the adolescent's feelings to communicate to him or her a sense of being understood, and thence a sense of being with someone who can be respected. At the same time, adolescents are particularly sensitive to any prying, and as with other age groups, the therapist needs to be careful about overintrusive interpretations and/or reflections. Thus for example, in the session (p. 164) when Patricia had been particularly angry with the therapist, it seemed clear that this was displaced anger which she was feeling towards her own family: interpreting this defence, however, would have created more anger, so after reflecting the fact that she was feeling angry, the therapist confined her response to a brief acknowledgement of what she herself was feeling.

Scrutinising and exploring the values of the adults with whom they come in close contact is very much a part of the process of developing an adult identity which is commonly seen as the major task of adolescence, even for those who do not experience the kinds of disjunctures to which Patricia was subjected; it is this developmental task which we consider in our next section.

THEORETICAL ISSUES

The development of adult identity

Developing a concept of self, a way of answering the question 'Who am I?', and of defining oneself and one's own sense of uniqueness in relation to others is a process which begins in infancy and arguably continues over the course of a lifetime. However, adolescence is regarded by Erikson and other developmental theorists as the period in which a stable, personal adult identity begins to be defined and established. This process of identity formation in adolescence is seen as one which incorporates yet transcends all previous conceptions of self. The self of childhood must give way to a sense of identity derived from, yet going beyond, these earlier foundations.

Many readers will be familiar with the framework in which Erikson delineates the emotional changes which occur at eight stages during the life span, and describes both the positive and negative potentials for each developmental stage. In adolescence, the task is to establish a sense of *identity*, and the negative pole, that of *role confusion*. Identity, as Erikson and others use the term, has multiple meanings, but is generally taken to be a composite of biological endowment, personal organisation of experience and cultural milieu. It can be described as a balance between that which is taken to be self and that considered to be other. The means by which we differentiate ourselves from other people in our lives as well as from our own organic functions constitutes the very core of our experiences of adolescent identity (Wilson et al., 1992).

During childhood, the mechanism of identification or 'being like' admired others, and assuming their roles and values is one of the primary means by which the child's sense of self is structured. Yet it is only on reaching adolescence that some of these childhood identifications can be selected and others discarded. This is in accordance with a more or less conscious recognition of the individual's interests, talents and values, and leads to the formation of an adult identity. It involves a synthesis of these earlier identifications into a new configuration, a process which is also crucially dependent on society's response.

With puberty, adolescents develop adult body size and shape, which brings, as well as a heightened self-awareness and a realisation of the body's new adult permanence, the emergence of new and powerful sexual feelings and emotions. Adult definitions of a sexual self, influenced by peers and the media, but also by family and their reactions to the emerging sexual identity, begin to be applied. Previous gender role training, as well as earlier relationships with the family, and with parents in particular, give guidelines for a new sexual identity, together with current gender role activities.

Shifting and powerful emotions, then, can emerge at adolescence which have remained dormant, or have even seemed resolved, at an earlier stage in childhood. Many examples from clinical experience show that as a child develops greater mental and emotional scope in adolescence, s/he may re-examine painful experiences and feel different and, on occasion, greater distress than when the event actually occurred. Pynoos and Eth describe, for example, an adolescent with whom they worked who:

> witnessed his mother's murder at the age of seven, but has only recently begun to focus on the possible significance of what he views as his mother's flirtatious behaviour. He now concludes that his mother was 'cheating' on her boyfriend and that this was the subject of the fatal argument. (1984: 96, quoted in our earlier book)

With a wide range of social interactions and greater freedoms, and the development of the capacity for complex abstract thought, the adolescent also begins to examine and question the roles, values and attributes of his or her parents. Adolescents may begin to test out and sift through parental characteristics and attitudes, reject, accept or modify them and sometimes develop mental strategies for changing themselves into the people they want to become.

We state above that adolescent identity is built on, but goes beyond the sense of self which has existed in childhood. This process of identity formation may incorporate the emotional tasks accomplished at earlier stages of development or highlight negative earlier experiences which need to be addressed. Following Erikson's framework, these emotional conflicts may emerge from the incomplete resolution of the four earlier developmental stages which involve the development of trust versus mistrust, autonomy versus shame and doubt, initiative versus guilt and industry versus inferiority.

Some, although not all, adolescents experience some kind of crisis in the process of trying to develop a stable and permanent sense of self. [See, for example, Marcia (1968) and Barker (1990) for a discussion of the different ways in which adolescents approach this task and their diverse responses to the 'turmoil' of adolescents. Barker, briefly reviewing the research, indicates that those showing psychiatric disorders in this age group are in a minority, and that even 'adolescent turmoil' was not evident in about two-thirds of the populations studied.] For Patricia, clearly, as for many adopted or fostered children, this process was made more difficult by a number of factors. Without adults to serve as a repository of memories from childhood, adolescents may feel inadequate or frustrated by having to rely completely on their own partial and incomplete memories. With Patricia this was compounded by a growing sense of being unable to trust what the significant adults said and the care that they had taken of her. So in much of her early work, she focused on issues of trust and mistrust, testing the therapist's trustworthiness, pouring scorn on the capacities of other adults outside her family circle who had been involved with her, contrasting this with her own family's consistency, and then gradually beginning to acknowledge that, in the pressure they placed on her to lie, and in their earlier abuse and/or failure to protect her, they had in fact shown themselves to be untrustworthy.

The process of separating from family, and rejecting some or all of their values and customs is painful and can produce, as it so clearly did for Patricia, feelings not only of confusion but loneliness – what do I stand for and believe in, if not the things my family stands for, and where do I belong, if not with them? Patricia's yearning to be back in her own bedroom, with her mother and with her own things, while at the same time recognising the real difficulties any such return would pose for her, was painful to witness.

However, at the same time as she began to dissociate herself from her family, she explored her relationships with her peers, and the growing importance that these friendships held for her, and the new self-confirming ways in which her girl friends supported her. Her relationships with the opposite sex were more problematic and, although this to some extent reflects a usual stage of adolescent exploration, this seemed an area which was incompletely addressed in her play therapy (a view confirmed in the account by Patricia's social worker later). Patricia herself clearly did not want to pursue it and there are several possible reasons for this. One possibility, of course, is that she was still preoccupied with her experiences of abuse from the adult males in her family, and too unsure of herself sexually to contemplate peer relationships with the opposite sex. It seems likely that she had not fully assimilated her abusive experiences and that her feelings of anger towards the abusers were displaced on to less powerful male figures. It is also possible that she did not feel safe or trustful enough of the therapist to discuss sexual experimenting fully with her, either because of her own inhibitions or her sense of inhibitions on the therapist's part. (Although we were not aware of this in reviewing the sessions, it is important to keep an open mind about the possibility that one may communicate unease at an unconscious level and also to be aware of social taboos which may inhibit an adolescent from discussing sexual encounters with someone from an older generation.)

Closely linked to these explorations was the beginning of the recognition, particularly in her relationship with her foster carer, Michael, that some adults were trustworthy, and could care for her in a loving and also altruistic way, so that she began to experience herself as a person lovable in her own right. Connected to this, too, was her attempt to understand and challenge the therapist's personality and values. Not only was this a significant process in testing out adult trustworthiness, but also it became part of differentiating who she was, her own feelings and experiences, from those of others, and seeing that differences could be acceptable rather than not permissable. Thus her pressure on the therapist to feel *the same* about her foster carer as she did had a quality of intensity which suggested that the exchange had considerable emotional significance for her. The therapist's firm assertion that her own relationship with Michael was different from Patricia's served the necessary purpose of acting as a counterpoint to her own relationship with him. In contrast to the blurring of boundaries which had been a hallmark of her family, she needed to see that the therapist's and, by implication, Sarah's relationship with Michael was different to her own. The therapist's clear sense of identity and values was, then, important, in helping her clarify different, appropriate family roles and boundaries.

The second stage of emotional development, autonomy versus shame and doubt, also emerged and was reworked in Patricia's therapy. Adolescents not only strongly desire autonomy in their personal lives, say in choosing clothes, friends and activities, but they also want to have the autonomy to develop their own set of values. Patricia's freedom to choose and act had been undermined, we would guess, within the family, giving her too much autonomy in some of her activities (for example, in the sexual abuse, or her freedom to dress in an older style) and not enough independence outside the family itself, as can be seen from her most decisive act, in divulging her abuse to someone outside the family, and the family's subsequent rejection of her because of this.

This self-direction is essential during adolescence. If an adolescent feels unduly pressured from others, s/he may feel unable to be their 'real' selves. In non-directive therapy, while the therapist still sets appropriate limits, these are broader than those with younger children, and the majority of decisions during the sessions are left to the adolescent, making the non-directive approach, we would argue, particularly well adapted to work with adolescents. Patricia's freedom, for example, to talk about personal issues, or not, as she wished, was made clear and respected, as were the limits of her behaviour. Of course, such issues, of the limits to autonomy and freedom, are always delicate ones in working with and caring for adolescents. They emerged for Patricia, without the therapist needing to act, when she divulged her dangerous activities. However, the therapist did need to weigh up and consult with others about her decision to end her therapy, and to balance Patricia's wishes in this respect with the therapist's recognition that some of her problems of anger and sexual conflicts with boys of her own age were probably a reflection of her earlier abuse and remained unresolved. Even more testing are those times, for example, when an adolescent's wish to return home, as Patricia did, or to live with one parent rather than another, is opposed by the therapist. Here the latter needs to have a firm sense of the appropriate limits to set to adolescent autonomy – an issue of course daily confronted by social work practitioners who must take into account, but also decide what weighting to give, the child or young person's wishes and feelings in any plans for their care.

In Patricia's explorations in therapy, then, can be seen a number of the processes involved in forming an adult sense of identity. These may involve the reworking of earlier stages of development, so that tasks, say, of expressing trust or autonomy have to be experienced and thought out in the context of new social situations, exercising greater choice, and in conjunction with increased intellectual capacity for reflection and analysis. Part of this process of identity formation involves scrutinising parental and family roles and values, and distancing oneself sufficiently from them to come to a balance for oneself by accepting some and rejecting others. Other adults are tested for possible role models (is this someone whom I respect and trust, whose values I like, and who I want to be like?), and the way in which others, particularly peers, react to the adolescent becomes an important determinant of his or her understanding of personal identity – the adult self-concept being, to some extent, the image which the self sees in a social mirror.

Where, as with Patricia, the family has in crucial ways been a damaging one, this process can be painful. Earlier stages may not have been healthily worked through, so that, for example, in an abusive family like hers, one can guess that the child's sense of initiative in forming relationships with those in authority might have been discouraged as being too threatening for the family's survival as a unit. Coupled with this, Patricia needed to find, as she moved away from her family, new relationships to confirm her in her sense of what she was becoming. Importantly, as we consider in the next section, her feelings about her sexuality needed to be addressed. Nonetheless, it is also possible through Patricia's therapy to understand why adolescence is seen (e.g. by Blos and others) to offer a 'second chance' and the opportunity to resolve earlier deficits and develop a positive and stronger sense of identity. There was, to us, something very moving and heartening in the strength of spirit and courage with which she faced the many changes in her young life.

The reworking of sexually abusive experiences in play therapy

A number of the other children we have written about in this book alleged, either before or during therapy, that they had been sexually abused, and we have briefly considered in these other chapters some practice issues related to these experiences, for example, issues of how to respond, how to set clear limits without letting the child feel shame or embarrassment, and issues of who else, if anyone, needs to be told and when. Here, we want to consider our theroretical understanding of the impact that sexual abuse has on the individual's sense of self, and the way in which non-directive play therapy addresses this impact. We have indicated that one aspect of the identity formation which is a major task of adolescence is the development of sexual identity and the adoption of adult sexual roles. It is therefore unsurprising that many adolescents who have been sexually abused experience extreme conflict and confusion over sexual roles and identity. Many children, too, who have been victims of abuse when younger, have renewed problems on reaching puberty. In Patricia's play therapy, she appeared to address these abusive experiences not only at a cognitive and emotional level, by exploring verbally her different reactions to what her step-father had done and expressing feelings about this, but also at a physical level, through moulding clay and coating and recoating her hands with paint. Although she verbalised her memories of disgust at the feelings engendered by having to masturbate her step-father, these verbalisations occurred separately from her work with the clay and paints, and consciously at least, she did not appear to connect the two. Similarly, Patricia never directly referred to her experience of sexual abuse by her uncle. This suggests the possibility that, although the experiences may have fused and been reworked symbolically, others may not have fully been brought into awareness at this point, and for Patricia might surface later.

In order to understand the distorting effects which sexual abuse has on the developing personality, its impact needs to be understood, as we suggested in our discussion of Diane's physical abuse in chapter 3, within a general framework of mental development. It involves responses at three different levels, the emotional, feeling level, the cognitive, intellectual level, and the motor or physical level (see Diane, chapter 3). In sexual abuse, strong, conflicting responses are engendered at all three levels. Thus, at the level of affect, the child may feel affection for the abuser but anger at being subjected to the abuse. Cognitively, she may consciously know that the act is wrong, but justify it as something that was not fully participated in. At a motor level, the abuse may produce sensations which are both painful and repellant yet pleasurable. Conflict may exist not only at each level but between levels, so that, for example, conscious awareness of the body's physical reaction is blocked out (i.e. dissociation).

These conflicts are very difficult for the child to assimilate into his or her existing schemas, since along with strong positive feelings towards carers, an attempt must also be made to assimilate equally or more powerful negative emotions which arise from the abuse. At a conscious level of awareness, the child may experience confusion and uncertainty, as when Patricia articulated the fact that some of the experiences with her step-father had been exciting, although scary. Many children, and this may have been the case with Patricia, although she did not directly say so, are also conscious of having found the experience physically arousing, while at the same time feeling that it is wrong or that they do not want it, and this too may give rise to feelings of guilt at having enjoyed it, and confusion at having done so.

Sexual abuse frequently engenders conflict on a motor level, since it commonly involves parts of the body and accompanying motor responses. The elementary motor schemas developed by a young child in relation to the body – for example, sucking as a baby, excretion, use of hands for exploration and manipulation – will be distorted by the sexual abuse. When parts of the body are misused and overstimulated, and especially if the abuse involves a family member (since a child's most basic schemas will have been developed through interactions with close family members), sexual abuse will affect relatively permanent and basic motor schemas and these schemas' interconnections with other basic affective and cognitive schemas. The child may feel dirty and helpless and, even if these feelings are openly acknowledged, s/he may not be able to integrate the motor activities in the abuse into existing motor schemas.

Patricia's play with clay and finger paints on her hands, turning them from the beautifully manicured objects from which she seemed slightly detached, into extremely messy ones which she coated over and over again, suggested the working through at a physical level of her past experiences. In making a mess of her own hands and then making them clean again, the sense of cleaning and purging herself came over very strongly. By doing this herself, she could begin to experience herself as in control rather than helpless and used as she had been during the act itself. Repeating this as she did over and over again, she seemed gradually able to set aside the sense of being powerless, and experience herself as someone who could own, and be in control of, her own bodily self, thus integrating her traumatic experiences into healthier schemas.

Her very specific reference to the unpleasant feelings she had had when having to masturbate her step-father lent credence to the hypothesis that this was an enactment of earlier experiences and ones that had involved this actual area of her body, i.e. her hands. With other children and adolescents, these reworkings of bodily experiences of abuse can be enacted at a symbolic level, with a more neutral or less private part of the body than was originally involved. Activities involving dolls or figures or sculptures may substitute for the actual, direct representation of what has occurred. In our earlier book (chapter 6), we gave examples of when a child made a penis out of playdough, or repeatedly inserted a hand and then an object into a lump of clay. Within a therapy session, the child can, as Patricia did, use some areas of the body that had been involved in sexual abuse, for instance the hands or the mouth, since it is socially acceptable to expose them. Other more intimate parts of the body which may have been directly involved in the abuse cannot be dealt with directly, because of social taboos, but may be represented symbolically.

The question of closeness to direct representation of the original act, or the extent of its transformation into a new symbol, before it can be recognised by the person as *representing* the abusive act symbolically rather than *disguising* it, is in our view incompletely resolved. With a non-directive approach, this question does not need to be resolved by the therapist, as the child will pick more or less disguised symbols, and choose to talk or not to talk. It becomes more of an issue in assessment, as the story of Ben demonstrates. Some of the work of Moore (Moore, 1995) on dreams, for example, suggests that the more an experience has been fully assimilated, the more likely it is to appear in dreams and in art symbolically rather than by direct representation. However, what exactly this process of assimilation consists of in particular is unclear. (See also Sinason's (1992) discussion of the way in which clients with severe learning disabilities need to have direct play experiences.)

As we point out in our earlier book, children play symbolically on different levels. At one extreme are symbols used in play that involve permanent, and basic affective and motor schemas. As we see with Patricia, symbolic play makes use of personal schemas embodying 'matters of intimate, permanent concerns, of secret and inexpressible desires' (Piaget, 1962: 175). At the other end of the continuum are objective schemas related to activities without hidden extra meanings.

Piaget gives an example of a child pretending he is a steeple. 'He is expressing what interests him in the widest sense of the word and there is certainly assimilation of reality to the ego. But these interests are only temporary' (1962:175). Although, as we have said earlier, this use of symbolic play diminishes in adolescence and in adulthood, we see in Patricia that it is by no means extinct; and the evidence of rituals and symbolic images in adult lives (the echoes of Lady Macbeth are powerful, of course) suggests an assimilative power remains.

The early sense which Patricia communicated, of her hands being rather separate from the rest of her, and with a life of their own, also suggested the kind of dissociative reaction which one frequently finds as a response to repeated abusive experiences. Although these are more usually described by those who have been abused as the feeling that the mind has left the body, it seems that sometimes one part of the body can be experienced as split off from the rest. An illuminating description of this bodily splitting due to trauma is to be found in Oliver Sachs' (1982) *A Leg to Stand On*, in which he describes the psychological aftermath of a severe injury to his leg, and his feeling that the leg was not part of him. He was helped through swimming to recover a complete sense of physical self. Patricia seemed to find her own solution to recovering her sense of completeness and gradually to be able to experience her hands as part of herself.

The therapist's responses during these episodes involving Patricia's hands were minimal, largely reflecting and articulating the latter's sensations and feelings, and acknowledged the change when Patricia began to allow the therapist to help. While the therapist should comment briefly on the child's symbolic play, in order to make it more conscious to the child, the latter does not necessarily need to talk, and is sometimes so immersed in the activity that verbalisation is minimal. It would of course have been possible to interpret these actions (as a psychoanalytic approach would suggest) to Patricia as enactments of the masturbation. This would, however, have run the risk of being too intrusive and threatening, by penetrating her mental defences against a highly anxious experience. A cognitive explanation also seemed unnecessary, and likely to deflect her from the feelings and sensations which were being resolved in the repeated covering of her hands.

This is not to say that links to traumatic past experiences should never be made. Often these experiences seem to be taking place on the very edge of consciousness, and the therapist is able to make an explicit link with a real event being half-remembered by the child. In other instances, the child may be half-remembering, confused, or misremembering an event, and the therapist is able to help the child with the correct facts, if aware of them. Sometimes, the symbolic enactment in therapy may be followed by an allegation, or a wish to talk about the experience, to others or to the child's or adolescent's carers. [See, for example, the case of Jeffrey in our earlier book (pp. 161–163) or Ben in this one.] This suggests a loosening of the child's defences and inhibitions, and the reduction of the child's own anxiety surrounding the event. The limited verbal descriptions offered by the therapist help the child re-integrate the trauma at a motor level. Having done so, the child is free to acknowledge what has happened cognitively and affectively as well.

To conclude, the impact of sexual abuse on a child involves motor responses and memories, as well as cognitive awareness and feelings, and it is important that the method of intervention adopted is capable of enabling the child to explore the experience on all three levels. Non-directive play therapy, because it utilises symbolic play rather than language alone, allows the child to express conflicts in a way which is appropriate to their own personal experience, and does not restrict this exploration to one particular level. With adolescents, more may be communicated at a verbal level, because of the greater verbal capacity of this age group, but the opportunity to work at a motor level is also provided when non-directive play therapy is employed.

We turn now to our final chapter. In this we consider a slightly different approach, that of using non-directive therapy for therapeutic assessments in court proceedings. We show how the approach can be adapted in order to help the court in making better-informed decisions on the child's welfare.

Chapter 7

Ben
A Therapeutic Assessment for the Court

*And to feel that the light is a rabbit-light
In which everything is meant for you
and nothing need be explained . . .
The trees are for you
The whole of the wilderness of night is for you,
A self that touches all edges . . .*
        Wallace Stevens 'A Rabbit as King of the Ghosts'

Non-directive play therapy as a method of assessment for the court is essentially a short-term, time-limited therapeutic intervention, which is conducted in the same manner as the longer term work with children we describe in our earlier chapters. However, there are particular issues in this type of work, which we illustrate in this concluding chapter through the story of Ben. We examine assessment issues more generally in the practice section, drawing out some of the differences and similarities to sustained therapeutic work with a child. Issues of particular concern, such as confidentiality, therapeutic suggestion, appropriateness and timing of assessments, and the writing of court reports based on play sessions will be explored. In the last section on theroretical issues we discuss ways in which the therapist distinguishes a child's wishes, feelings and fantasies from real current and past events in the child's life.

BACKGROUND INFORMATION

I first learned about Benjamin when his guardian *ad litem*, Raymond, asked me whether I would conduct an assessment of him for the court. Ben was a nine year old who was in the care of the local authority on an Interim Care Order and had now been living with foster parents for about three months. He had previously been living on his own with his father, Robert Jones, who had had sole parental responsibility for him since his mother had disappeared when he was four years old. She had eventually been traced to London, where she was living with a new partner, and had decided to sever her ties with everyone, including Ben, in the north.

The local authority had had concerns about Ben's parenting and his poor care for some time. More recently, he had developed a close relationship with his male teacher and had begun to relate to him incidents which appeared to be of an emotionally abusive nature. Social workers had tried to work cooperatively with Ben's father, but these incidents had increased in frequency and severity. Ben appeared to be at risk of significant harm both emotionally and physically and Ben himself was beset by abnormal fears and a general nervousness. The local authority felt they had no recourse other than to apply for a Care Order on him.

Raymond thought that a non-directive approach could be beneficial for Ben because, since his removal from home, he had been extremely reluctant to talk to any professionals. Raymond had visited him at his foster home and had tried to talk very generally with him while his foster carers, Pam and Daniel, had been present, but Ben had seemed so nervous and withdrawn that he had desisted. Since direct work appeared to be too threatening to him, perhaps I might be able to help Ben express his needs, wishes and feelings indirectly through play. I would then also be in a position to give an opinion on his future therapeutic needs to the court. In the mean time, Raymond would continue his interviews with Ben's father and mother. No other extended family members had been identified as possible future carers for Ben so Raymond intended to confine his interviews to the parents, other professionals involved with the case and to reading the social services file. Raymond also told me that Mr Jones' solicitor had asked for an assessment for his client from another psychologist. Raymond intended to meet this psychologist later.

A non-directive approach seemed to me an appropriate way of assessing Ben. Also since the final court hearing was four months away, and the time-scale for this kind of assessment was approximately nine weeks, my work could realistically be completed in time. Raymond and I agreed to meet again in about seven weeks, when our assessments would both be nearing completion.

Following my appointment as an expert witness at a directions hearing that week and the release of papers in the proceedings to me by the court for the purpose of preparing a report, the solicitor applied for my funding to the Legal Aid Board. After another week I received a letter from her, the 'letter of instruction', which formed part of the documentary evidence in Ben's case and would be included in the bundle of documents for court use. This letter formally stated, amongst other things, that the aim of my assessment at the request of the guardian was to identify whether Ben showed signs of behavioural difficulties and, if so, whether these difficulties were due to inappropriate parenting. Further questions concerned Ben's longer term needs, evidence of his own wishes and feelings concerning his father, and whether his future needs could be met by remaining with his father.

I also received court documents with the solicitor's letter, which consisted of statements filed by the local authority for the preliminary hearing. As an expert in Ben's case, I depended upon the solicitor for receiving the relevant documentation in the case. (However, it was my duty as an expert to request additional information or documentation from her, if the information I had received seemed incomplete.) Ben's solicitor, acting on instructions from the guardian, was specialised in childcare law and a member of the Childcare Panel of the Law Society. She would therefore know in general what documents the expert would need initially and as the case proceeded, but might not know an expert's more specific requirements. (When the therapist is instructed by the solicitor for a child's parent or carer, rather than the guardian or local authority, the solicitor may not be a member of the panel and may be less experienced in childcare cases. The expert needs to be even more alert in these cases to the possibility that the documentation is incomplete.)

The documents in Ben's case gave me the name of the key social worker, Lynn, and her summary of his background history. Lynn had described the work undertaken with Ben's father, and included the written contracts between him and the local authority for changes needed in his care of Ben. An assessment by the family centre staff of Ben's parenting and a family chronology were also given. Lynn's statement gave the immediate reasons for Ben's removal from home. Ben had alleged to his teacher that his Dad had dragged him out of the house and locked him in the garden shed for the night. He had seemed extremely nervous during the joint investigation into his allegation, and would not say any more. He did say to Lynn on the way to his foster carers that he didn't want to go home, saying that his dad would 'kill' him for talking behind his back. Her report outlined previous social services involvement when his mother had left and his father had taken over his care, and an investigation two years ago into a report by a neighbour that Ben was screaming on most nights so loudly that they could hear him easily through their walls. No evidence of physical abuse had been found and Ben's father attributed Ben's behaviour to nightmares.

My subsequent meeting with Lynn was an opportunity to supplement information I had already received from the court. Raymond would be interviewing Ben's teacher and I arranged with Lynn to send me all his school reports. Lynn reported that Ben was generally withdrawn and timid at school, of low average intelligence and sometimes seemed to find it difficult to concentrate on his work. His general appearance had been scruffy; he still had poor personal cleanliness and grooming. His relationships with other children were not good – he tended to remain on the outside of groups of boys without being able to join in their activities. Occasionally he would team up with a very aggressive boy in his class and tease children in the youngest classes.

Lynn also gave me more details of his allegation. On the day he had alleged abuse, his teacher, Mr Blackburn, had asked him why he wasn't wearing a jacket, because the weather had turned quite cold overnight. Ben had told him about his night in the shed spontaneously, then had appeared very frightened and beside himself, saying frantically that he didn't want to say that and not to tell his dad. His teacher had needed to spend quite a while calming him down and telling him gently that teachers had to tell other people who protected children when they were badly treated, but he would also tell them what Ben had said about his dad knowing he had told. Lynn added that they had managed to find Ben an emergency foster placement and then his current placement nearer to his school, and he was still in Mr Blackburn's class. His relationship with his teacher had become if anything a bit closer since Ben had lived at his foster home.

Long-term fostering at his current placement was proposed as Ben's future care plan, but the local authority was uncertain what contact with his father he needed and were waiting for more information, including my report, before deciding what to propose. The contact visits between Ben and his father were currently once a week, supervised by a staff member. Sometimes these visits went well: Ben and his father were physically affectionate with one another, and got involved in playing board games and energetic football games together. However, at other times the contacts did not work so well: Ben seemed wary and distant, and his father seemed preoccupied with talking to the worker and virtually ignored Ben. The staff member could not pinpoint what caused this difference, but the atmosphere of the sessions was very obvious. Perhaps if these contact visits were maintained, but not held so frequently, they might be a better experience for Ben. I asked to have access to all current and future recorded contact notes in order to think about this issue.

Lynn went on to say that she did not feel that she herself had any rapport with Ben. She had seen him numerous times and always tried to make him smile and relax in her presence, but he remained wooden and serious, and was monosyllabic in his answers. When she visited him in his foster home, Ben stayed near her as little as possible and tried never to be alone with her. Lynn was very worried about him because he was so distant and withdrawn.

I had a lengthy, preparatory discussion about Ben with Lynn and his foster carers; we discussed my method of working and aspects of Ben's behaviour which worried them. They found it unusual that Ben never directly mentioned home or his dad to them; but sometimes he seemed to let his guard down and something slipped out. They had noted these down in their diary notes. For example, last week Ben had been absorbed in a TV programme and saw a man with a lasso. He blurted out that the rope was like the one his dad had tied him up with once, but longer. Then he had become panic-stricken, shouted that he had never said that, and ran away to hide in the bathroom. Another time he talked about the food he was eating as much better than dog biscuits in a very matter-of-fact manner. They had also observed and recorded that Ben's night-time enuresis and nightmares were lessening, but seemed to happen regularly before and after his contacts with his dad.

We talked further about Ben's relationships with them and with the other children in their family. In the first month or so, Pam and Daniel were agreed that Ben kept to himself and was silent and withdrawn. Very recently, he seemed more settled into their home and to be playing more with the other children. He had started to talk to them about the other children and was beginning to want their individual attention.

I arranged to come to their house in order to introduce myself to Ben later in the week. My final preparation before beginning his therapeutic assessment was to arrange to see Ben's father at a family centre near his house, writing to him to introduce myself, and explaining briefly what I would be doing and what I was hoping to talk with him about. I made the appointment for two weeks' time, in order to have started sessions with Ben and to have a better idea from knowing him personally what Ben was like.

BEN'S PLAY THERAPY SESSIONS

Ben's play therapy

Ben entered the playroom with Pam, eyes downcast, and sat on the armchair on the far side of the room with Pam next to him, while I went to sit on a lower chair midway between Ben and the door. Pam said that she had talked with Ben about coming here and waiting for him while he played. I briefly spoke to him about the length of our sessions and the number of times I had planned that we would be together. I repeated that Raymond had asked me to see him and write some things for the judge to decide what Ben needed about his father. If Ben wanted me to, we could talk later on, after we knew one another better, about what I was going to write. Ben remained silent, looking at the floor. I quietly remarked that maybe he didn't know what to make of all this, and that he was waiting to find out what would happen to him. Because he had avoided me when I'd come to introduce myself earlier, I added that I didn't ask a lot of questions of children when they came to the playroom; Ben could play or talk, or do what he wanted more or less when we were together. I saw children here who were troubled about some things or who had difficult things happening to them. Some of them were quiet with me, just like Ben was being now.

Ben continued to look down as I finished talking, but shifted his gaze to the left fractionally, spotted a soft sponge ball near him and reached out for it, then began tossing it in front of him, keeping his eye fixed deliberately on the ball's movements and away from myself. There was a pause, a silence and Pam signalled to me with her eyes that she intended to leave. I slightly nodded to her and she asked Ben if he was all right, then? Ben's attention remained riveted on the ball and Pam rose from her chair, saying that she'd be in the waiting room next door. Ben sighed a small sigh and Pam left. Once alone with me, Ben redoubled his efforts, throwing the ball higher and faster than before.

I confined my remarks to the ball, saying that Ben seemed interested in how fast and high he could make it go. Several minutes passed; I remained interested in what Ben was doing and made a few brief remarks to him about his actions. Then Ben seemed deliberately to throw the ball out of reach and watched the ball roll towards me. I smiled, saying that now I could help him and threw the ball back to him. Ben glanced at me briefly from time to time after this as he continued to toss the ball in front of him. Then he let the ball drop near the blackboard at his end of the room and glanced at the chalk, then fleetingly at me. I responded that all the things in the room were for him to use and that maybe he was finished with the ball for now and wanted to use the blackboard.

Ben turned his back to me and began to write on the board. First he wrote his name Ben over and over around the periphery of the board, then he concentrated on writing 'Ben Jones' in capital letters in the middle of the board, going over the individual letters several times in different coloured chalks. I watched, talking briefly about how important his name was to him, and that now I knew his name very well, too. I had read some things about him and now I was getting to know him. Ben admired his work, then added the names of his foster carers, Pam and Daniel, beneath his own name. I again remarked that they seemed important to him and he was putting them close to his own name.

Ben rubbed out all his writing, then sat half-turned towards me and looked around the room, then at the board again. I said 'Wondering whether you're finished with that yet?' Ben turned towards the board again and began to draw a cartoon figure of a man, full front, with a big nose and spikey hair. He quickly drew small circles and shaded them in (which I thought to myself resembled holes) on the man's forehead, chest and arms.

V: Maybe there's something wrong with him?
B: [*sotto voce*] Bang! Bang! He's dead! Sixty bullets in his head!
V: Playing that he's VERY dead, holes everywhere in that man!

Ben then very deliberately drew crosshatches over the cartoon until the man disappeared, and I commented that he wanted to get rid of it so that no one could see the dead man. Ben wrote his name again, and the address of his foster home. I commented that Ben wasn't thinking of the dead man anymore; he was back to thinking about himself now and where he lived.

Leaving this message on the blackboard, Ben returned to the sponge ball. He stood up and began to toss the ball into the air, then positioned himself underneath and kicked the ball off the heel of his right foot. I commented, as I took in his exertions, that it didn't look easy! He must need to practise to do that. Ben told me in a strained voice, with his eye remaining on the ball as he continued to kick, that he had football skills practice with Mr Blackburn today in PE. I replied, 'It looks like that's something you look forward to a lot'. Ben nodded in the direction of the ball and continued to practise, then asked me if I'd count his kicks. I counted and commented that Ben wanted both of us to know when he'd done a lot. Ben was getting fewer and fewer kicks in a running sequence as he doggedly continued.

V: You don't want to give up. It's something you want to be very good at doing... You can't kick it as well now, but you still don't want to stop...
[Ben then asked me if I wanted a go.]
V: Yes, sure. Maybe you're thinking you could have a rest when I have a go. You don't have to do all the work then!

Ben collapsed onto the beanbag on the side of the room, watching me with the ball. I tried to imitate Ben's technique, but gave a very poor performance. I laughed at myself, saying that I wasn't as young or as good at football as Ben was. Ben gave a secret smile, then began to laugh outright as I made a renewed effort to connect my heel with the ball.

B: That's not the way! It's like this [as he came up to me and took over the ball]. Now it's your turn.

We spent the remainder of the hour with Ben practising his skills and intermittently having me practise my very rudimentary ones. He returned to Pam, telling her that it had been fun and that we had played football.

Ben's next two sessions fit the pattern he had devised in our first hour. He spent the first part of the second session at what seemed to be an emotionally deep level and the rest of the time being physically very active playing football, sometimes on his own and sometimes including me. In his third session, Ben decided to paint for the first part of the hour. He began by painting a brown house with a path up to the door and a small garden in the front with bushes near the path. The windows were outlined in green and the front door was green as well. I said 'That house looks familiar. I wonder if it's Pam and Daniel's?' Ben nodded and asked me to put it up to dry because he wanted to bring it home.

As I took it from him, he took another sheet of paper and told me that it was going to be another house. He started to do the outline this time in black – black windows and door were added, and then he layered more and more black paint on to the sky, muttering about the cold, and becoming very intense and silent as he worked.

> V: Everything is looking so cold and dark outside. The house is very black and dark, seeing it from the outside. Nothing seems to be moving in the house or outside in the dark. [As Ben layered more paint on] It's so dark outside that you can almost feel the darkness, it's so thick. And it's everywhere, you can't get away from it . . . [I felt a growing sense of oppression and desperation as he worked on the darkness in his painting.]

Ben remained silent, but abruptly started making black lines crosshatching the house, then began gouging the damp paper with his brush. I said 'Wanting it to be destroyed. You want to ruin it and get rid of it.' Ben shoved the whole house into the dustbin savagely and went to wash his hands. I offered to get the nailbrush for him when I saw him struggling with the paint on his hands, and talked to him about how hard it was to get rid of the black once it was on so thickly.

Once more we played football for the remainder of the hour, this time keeping score of our kicks for our favourite teams. His team scored very well and mine came a poor second. As we played, I commented on how much he liked to be good at football and think about how the professional players do it. Maybe he liked to pretend that he was on their team when he was practising. Ben said that he did and that he pretended that he was Gary Lineker. Who was I going to be? I mentioned 'Gazza', but Ben thought that I should be someone else because 'Gazza' was a 'crybaby'. (This was just after the World Cup game in which Paul Gascoigne had cried on the pitch when penalised and been barred from playing in the final.) I said 'I don't mind if men cry when they're upset. But if it worries you, I can be someone else.' Ben nodded and had me 'be Bryan Robson instead'.

With about fifteen minutes left of our session, I told Ben that I was planning to see his father in a few days' time. I was going to tell him in general about what I did with children who came to the playroom. I said I was going to talk about what his Dad thought was best for Ben, but not about what Ben and I did together. I'd leave that up to Ben to talk to people about, except for the reports I had to write at the end. I noticed that Ben had a glazed look coming over his face as I talked and he began hurriedly to toss the ball in the air in front of him. I asked him if he wanted to hear any more about it and he shook his head slightly, immediately telling me to kick the ball between our pretend goal. For the rest of the time we played football without talking about anything except the game itself.

Meeting Ben's father

My meeting with Mr Jones at the family centre started with an explanation to him of my method of working with children in non-directive play therapy and my instructions from Raymond, Ben's guardian. Mr Jones spent considerable time giving me details of Ben's mother's departure and the difficulties he had being a single parent. I acknowledged these difficulties, especially for a man, in finding a strong support system to help him with Ben's care. Mr Jones refuted the need for 'interference', as he labelled it, saying that he'd already had too much of that from social services. He'd be fine if they'd let him 'get on with it'. I tried to bring our conversation around to Ben several times, but did not successfully get him to concentrate on what Ben needed as a nine-year-old boy and how these needs were different to his own. Mr Jones did discuss the good times they had together and accused social services of trying to run him down to everyone.

He then began to talk about Ben needing firmness, that he was far too cheeky, and that his way of dealing with Ben had been good enough for him when he was a lad and was good enough for Ben. We discussed Mr Jones' methods of disciplining Ben, which sounded highly punitive to me for minor misdemeanors. When I suggested that there were other milder methods more in keeping with Ben's behaviour, Mr Jones became indignant, accusing me angrily of not being able to help him or understand him. I suggested that my job had been to get to know Ben and what Ben needed, and that I did want to find those things out from Mr Jones' point of view. I suggested that he work with the psychologist who was undertaking an assessment of him for the court, where he could concentrate on important issues for himself and for Ben. We agreed to finish on that note.

Ben's middle sessions

For our next session Ben came in looking very pleased with his appearance, wearing new tracksuit bottoms, a new team strip and new trainers. He stopped inside the door to the room and made a point of tying the lace of his new trainer. I remarked that Ben seemed proud of his new things and wanted to take care of them well. He smiled into the space in front of him as he finished tying his lace, then walked very deliberately and confidently over to the monsters at the far end of the room. There were three to choose from – a brown one with lines meant to resemble hair covering its body, upright and with near-human features; a soft, flexible dinosaur made out of stuffed nylon material, with a long stiff tail; and a dark green plastic monster with deformed body and limbs, sharp fangs in a large, gaping mouth and claw-like extremities. Ben picked this last one, the fiercest one, and went through very aggressive, intense and prolonged play sequences with it as he pretended to destroy it – he shot at it with a popgun, dropped it down a 'hole', stabbed it and finally went into very close range and kicked the monster repeatedly in the head. I reflected his feelings verbally with a fierceness in my tone of voice, saying that he wanted above all to destroy it, but that it was too hard for him to do. He had to keep at it and it still didn't go away. I reflected how he had to use such awful ways to hurt it and seemed to be trying to make it leave him alone. Ben stopped kicking the monster and calmed down as I spoke about these feelings. He then said that he'd had enough of that and it was time to play football again.

As we played, Ben talked about his school football team, and how he and his friend were practising a lot, hoping they'd get really good. We talked about his hope of getting good enough to try out for the team, and Ben went through with me all the football skills he knew, having me try them out and being very patient with me when I was inevitably inept. I commented on how I was able to keep trying when he was so nice to me and remarked later that I didn't feel foolish when I couldn't do things because he didn't laugh at me. He just tried his best to help me.

When I walked out with him at the end of the hour to where Pam was waiting, she asked me whether Ben had mentioned that he had a school trip next week that he wanted to go on. I shook my head, but said to Ben that it was fine by me and that we could either make up the time or skip it out, whichever he wanted to do. Ben said 'Skip it', in a barely audible voice, and I replied that maybe Ben was worried about what I might say, but that it was up to him and we would have two more times before we finished, then Ben nodded, relieved, and went off cheerfully.

Lynn, Ben's social worker, telephoned me a few days later to let me know that Ben had told Pam that he didn't want to see his father this week. When Lynn went to talk to him, Ben had said to her that he wanted to go to soccer practice after school. Ben's father, however, had reacted very badly, becoming enraged and saying that his son had been 'brainwashed' by Lynn, Pam and Daniel, and myself. He also threatened not to attend the visits with Ben any more if that was the way Ben was going to treat him. Lynn, knowing that Ben had decided not to have one of his sessions with me, wondered if the two were related. I told Lynn that children who come to play therapy sessions do often tend to gain a clearer sense of what they want and that, when children do assert their independence appropriately, it was quite important for the adults to adapt their behaviour as well. Also, as she knew, football obviously meant a lot to children his age. It was a way boys in particular were able to show their competence and to interact positively with their peers. I saw it as very positive that Ben seemed to feel confident enough with her that he could assert his choice clearly. Lynn pointed out that she had mentioned to Ben that his father would be disappointed, but Ben hadn't wavered. He had just retreated as soon as he could to play outside with the other children. Lynn added that future contact sessions would be closely monitored to see whether Ben's need to see his father was changing and how his father would react to what he seemed to view as an act of disloyalty towards himself on Ben's part. I wrote notes as Lynn talked, remembering that, in the contact notes of Ben's visits with his father, the supervisor had noted that Ben never made suggestions himself or objected to what his father decided.

Ben came to his next session and walked easily into the playroom, picking up the sponge ball to toss into the air as he went past it. After standing in the middle of the room for a while, nonchalantly tossing the ball into the air and kicking it with his heel, he turned directly towards me and said that he might do something different today. He took the toy dinosaur and had me hold it, then took the green monster himself and enacted a story in which the dinosaur gets into trouble for pinching some food from the monster, then runs away and hides while the monster rages because the dinosaur is out of sight. We played out all these actions, with Ben directing my movements. I verbalised the dinosaur's hunger and fear of the monster after checking out with Ben what he wanted the dinosaur to feel. Ben was very animated and immersed in the story, engaged in the action in a way that he had not been before. After having several goes at variations on this scene, with the dinosaur trying out different hiding places and different ways of placating the monster, Ben decided to enlist the help of the hand puppets in the room. He had the fox, which he portrayed as cunning and wily, steal the food and leave some pretend food in the dish. Then the bird carried the dinosaur up into the sky and away from the fierce monster, waiting until everything was silent and still down below before returning to earth with the dinosaur again. (Ben performed all the voices of the animals, while my role devolved into being the narrator of the feelings and thoughts of the characters. Ben's smooth actions and 'flow' seemed to show that my comments followed his story well, without interrupting the evolution of his story, which seemed emotionally creative and meaningful for him.)

Most of our hour was spent in this extended story about the dinosaur's adventures, his eventual return to earth and his play with the friends who had helped him get food and escape. All the creatures finished their adventure by being treated to watching a football match, with Ben as the star player. I became one of the spectators, cheering when goals were made and 'talking' with the other creatures about how pleased we were that Ben was enjoying himself so much and doing so well at this game. I also mentioned how pleased his team was to have him with them and scoring for them against the other team. Ben finished and ran to tell Pam about our game, exuberantly telling her that he'd 'had a great time with Virginia today and scored all the goals himself'.

Progress meeting with Ben's guardian *ad litem*

Before my last meeting with Ben I had scheduled a meeting with Raymond, Ben's guardian, to exchange information about our separate work. I began by saying that, in my opinion, Ben had altered considerably in a short time. He seemed to have changed from a very introverted, fearful boy with low self-esteem to a boy who was much more extroverted and confident of himself. This change did not seem to be confined to his behaviour within our sessions and to his increased familiarity with me and with the sessions, but seemed to extend to his relationship with Lynn, with his peers and even with his father. Raymond confirmed that in his meeting with Ben's teacher, Mr Blackburn had remarked on how noticeable the positive changes in Ben were at school since his move into foster care. He was able to concentrate on his school work better, he spontaneously participated in class more often and he certainly was beginning to make new friends with boys in his class. Ben seemed more ready to approach other staff members now, and in general was more presentable and more cheerful.

Ben's foster carers had reported that his enuresis was more or less over with, and that he was taking a real pride in his appearance. He also was more happy with both of them and sought out their company. Ben wanted Daniel to be involved with his school football activities and Pam to listen to his home reading every night. He was also beginning to unthaw in his feelings, and would laugh and become boisterous more readily, scowl and answer back and let them hug him more easily. His nightmares did still trouble him at times, though, but he seemed able to call out to them and then be reassured, leaving his light on to help him get back to sleep.

I discussed the themes from Ben's play sessions, which seemed to centre on developing age-appropriate skills, the gradual development of trust in my help and goodwill towards him, and the extreme fearfulness and hate he played out which were likely to be related to his earlier experiences with his father. He had not yet been able to relate these highly negative feelings directly himself to his real-life experiences, or talk directly about his wishes and feelings concerning his father. I thought it evident from the quantity and highly charged quality of these emotions that they had affected his emotional development adversely.

I also discussed with Raymond the meeting I had had with Mr Jones, and his inability when with me to concentrate on Ben's needs or on how he could change his attitudes and behaviour to meet these needs. I had been struck by Mr Jones' negative reaction to Ben's desire to attend football practice and skip their contact. Ben might be concerned he would be punished in some way emotionally for his father's disappointment, which could explain his overcompliance at contact visits. Ben's behaviour during contacts also fitted in well with research evidence on patterns of passivity and compliance in children abused by carers over a more lengthy period of time. (See Diane, chapter 3.)

Raymond mentioned that he had observed a contact visit between Ben and his father. In this visit, which was after Ben had not seen his father because of football practice, Ben seemed to go out of his way to placate his father and to please him. He constantly checked on what his father wanted to do and if what they were doing was enjoyable to him. While Mr Jones was participating in activities where he was winning, such as draughts, his interactions with Ben were reasonable, but if the tables turned and Ben was beginning to win or was getting restive with his father always winning, as he did late on in the contact, Mr Jones became very irritated and impatient, saying that they might as well end their time early since Ben was so fed up with things. Ben then immediately shifted activities to suit his father and they once again got along reasonably together.

We discussed our joint need for the conclusions of Mr Jones' psychological assessment, which was not yet finished. With the information we had to date, we agreed, Mr Jones' prognosis for change to meet Ben's developmental needs was not very likely, but we would await the report. Finally, we discussed whether weekly contact with his father was too emotionally demanding for Ben. I felt that as Ben seemed to be increasingly able to make up his own mind, the way forward might be to leave visits up to the discretion of the local authority, in order to adjust to Ben's changing needs. We would need to check the local authority's view on this proposal and how they would implement it in practice.

Ben's last session

At the beginning of our last session, I reminded Ben that I had offered to tell him about what I was going to write to the judge. Did he want to know? Ben shook his head forcefully, without speaking. I said 'You're very sure you don't want to hear anything. That's all right with me.' Ben again retreated into tossing the sponge ball around for a bit, then said that I was to pretend that I was being sent out to play.

V: Maybe I'm a child, then.
B: Right! I send you out to play . . . You kick a ball into a garden and break sommat.
B: Take your ball and get out to play.
V: Bye, . . . what do I call you?
B: Dad.
V: Bye, Dad. See you later. [To myself] I'll lark around here . . . Wonder how high I can kick it? [I give the ball a hard kick] CRASH! Oh, my God! What'll I do? [running around frantically in circles and looking over my shoulder]
B: You run and hide and don't go back home till late.
V: [hiding behind some beanbags] Maybe everybody'll forget what happened if I clear out.
B: Say 'I'll get a good hiding if me dad catches me'. [V repeats in a frightened voice].
B: You crawl out and sneak in the house but I catch you and whop you.
V: [when creeping around the room] I hope I can just get into my bed before he catches me . . .
B: [yelling and turning the light switch on and off] Get over here! Get your shoe off and hand it to me!
V: [aside] Do I do everything you tell me or not?
B: [aside] EVERYTHING!
V: I'm so scared. Here's my shoe. [cowering]
B: Say 'Sir' and CRAWL!
V: [crawling carefully] Yes, sir.
B: [hitting the shoe rhythmically on the palm of his hand] I know what! I'll lock you outside. Then I can come to get you ANYTIME I want! [slapping the shoe hard against the wall]
V: [starting in alarm at the slap on the wall and flinching] [Aside] What do I do next?
B: You cry and ask me to let you stay where it's warm, but I don't.
V: [crying] I'll do anything you want, but don't make me go outside!
B: I don't care how cold you get, you smelly fart. [pretending to drag me out] Stay shut up there until I come for you. And then you'll see how your arse can hurt!
[V starts quivering and submits. B looks extremely anxious and pauses]
B: [changing to an excited tone] Then you crash the door down in the shed, go out and find all the . . . Wait! I'll be the boy and you can be the dad. I'm finding all the big dogs you can hear howling and barking in the night and let them in the house! No, you help me. [using the large stuffed toys] We'll get all the dogs! Come on! And we get him. We'll tear him to bits!
V: We're so cold and scared. We want to hurt him, to stop him from

hurting us.
B: Yeah! [throwing toys into the designated house area]

I join in and we laugh excitedly together as we throw the toys one after the other into the 'house'. Ben then collapses in exhaustion onto a beanbag and I join him. He smiles and then laughs freely, with a sense of relief in his tone of voice. Gradually becoming relaxed and thoughtful, Ben says he wants to make me something before he goes. Getting a large piece of paper, he folds it into a card shape, draws a large house on the front in red, green and yellow and writes inside (asking me how to spell my name):

To Virginia   From your frend   Ben.

He decided to leave a few minutes early to return to Pam. I thanked both of them for coming and told Ben that I would miss our time together. Then I returned thoughtfully to the playroom to tidy up, preoccupied with all that had happened in our last session.

I was concerned that Ben would probably have benefited from more sessions with me immediately, rather than having to wait for more funding to be allocated to my independent practice by the local authority. If this funding was not made available, as was all too frequently the case due to scarce resources, Ben then would be required to start anew with another therapist in the community health service. When his name eventually rose to the top of their waiting list, the service may or may not identify this type of intervention as suitable in their opinion for his therapeutic needs. An additional problem could arise in their lack of staff trained and supervised in non-directive play therapy. I was left with my mixed feelings of satisfaction in having helped Ben and having conducted a useful assessment, in my opinion, for the court, along with a sense of disappointment primarily for Ben, but also personally, in leaving his life at this juncture, an issue I decided to earmark for my next consultation supervision.

BEN'S COURT REPORT

I began my report by listing my qualifications, including my experience in working in statutory settings and my special interest in non-directive play therapy, the source of my instructions, the aim of my assessment, and the sources of information for my report, which included my meetings and the documents I had read in preparing my report.

I explained the non-directive play therapy method of assessment I used with Ben, including my method of recording our sessions. I then described Ben, beginning with the way he presented himself at the outset of our work together:

> Ben was unusually withdrawn and seemed very apprehensive of me in our introductory meeting, and at the beginning of our first session. As he began to relax emotionally within our sessions, Ben became more extroverted and assertive; he began to play out his strong aggressive feelings, which seemed more intense than usual for his chronological age. He also began to demonstrate a more positive self-image as our sessions progressed; his appearance improved and he developed competence and closer peer relationships, which were more normal for his chronological age. Ben appeared to be of average intelligence and his fine and large physical skills seemed normal for his age.

The report next considered Ben's play therapy sessions, first setting out their contents, organised into three themes, which were emotionally important to Ben during the sessions, and then commenting on these and giving my recommendations in the light of these and other information about him.

Themes reported in Ben's play sessions

Aggression and fearfulness

In Ben's early sessions he showed a very high level of aggression when drawing a cartoon figure of a man and in his play with a toy monster. As our sessions progressed, his aggression became incorporated into role-plays of a figure that was in trouble with the monster, needing to placate it and then hide from it. In our last session Ben's role-play was specifically about a 'Dad' who threatened a child with severe punishment. The child was extremely fearful of the father and was tormented by him; the child then became aggressive towards the father in turn.

The development of a more positive self-concept

Ben's aggressive and fearful play described above was in marked contrast to his other positive feelings and play. He drew two houses, for example, with one resembling his foster home, which was depicted as attractive and pleasant, while the other was a dark, cold house which he destroyed when he had finished painting it. He also took increasing pride in his appearance as our sessions continued and was increasingly interested in developing his school-related sports skills. Ben mentioned a friend at school, and was able to be patient and understanding in a helping role with me. Ben also became more assertive in our sessions;

for example, he was able to state that he wanted to cancel one of our sessions because of another outside activity at school. He was also able spontaneously to express positive feelings towards me by the end of our time together.

Ben's attachments

While Ben did not discuss his feelings directly concerning his attachments in our sessions together, he did become more spontaneous and expressive with his foster carer, Mrs Robinson, who brought him to the sessions, as our sessions progressed. He also wrote out his foster carers' names near his own and drew their house, as stated above. Ben mentioned his teacher, Mr Blackburn, once in a positive way. He did not, however, speak about his father directly in any of our sessions. When his father was mentioned by me before my own meeting with Mr Jones, and again when I mentioned my court report concerning Ben's needs about his father in our first and last sessions, Ben seemed to become very withdrawn and uncomfortable with this topic. Ben played out the scene described above in which a father figure used intimidation, threats and physical punishment after the child had accidently broken something, then confining his child to a shed late at night in the cold. The scene, as discussed below, seemed to be directly related to a very abusive event Ben had experienced earlier with his father. He did not directly or indirectly mention his mother in our sessions, nor did any of his play sequences involve a maternal figure.

Comments on Ben's play themes

Ben's emotional development, in my opinion, appears to have been damaged by his experiences while in the care of his father. The aggression and fearfulness he expressed in his play was at first vague, involving a powerful (probably male) figure, and then became centred on a father figure who treated him with cruelty. These themes in his play therapy sessions corresponded to the information available to me from professionals in preparing this report. In particular, Ben's role-play of a child being severely punished by being locked in the shed for the night by the father fitted the information he gave to his teacher earlier about his treatment by his father. It is likely, in my opinion, that Ben was re-enacting his own traumatic experience in the role-play; his emotions were appropriate to the scene and very highly charged, with emotional exhaustion after this scene. He also changed the role-play in a way that is described in the psychological literature on traumatised children, denoting a healing process; that is, he himself took the role of the abusive father, then joined with me in a fantasy destruction of this powerful paternal figure (see Pynoos and Eth, 1984; Gil 1991). As well as the positive changes in Ben's self-esteem within our sessions and his increased emotional relaxation with me, Ben seemed to be beginning to be more assertive in stating his wishes to his social worker regarding contacts with his father. He also seemed to be indicating that he was developing closer attachments to his foster carers and developing positive relationships at his school with both staff and peers.

Recommendations

1. Ben's needs seem well met in his current foster placement and he seemed to be indicating indirectly in his sessions that his wish is to remain with them. While I have not had the benefit of the psychologist's report on Mr Jones in preparing my report, and I may revise my opinion in light of its conclusions, from my own meeting with Mr Jones it seemed unlikely that his attitudes towards Ben's parenting would change sufficiently within the time-scale needed by Ben for rehabilitation to his father's care. Due to his emotional damage from earlier experiences, Ben needs more sensitive, sustained and supportive parenting than normal, which his foster carers seem able to give him. In my opinion, and in the light of my current information, Ben's needs seem best met in a secure, long-term foster placement with Mr and Mrs Robinson, leading to a later consideration of a Residence Order to further stabilise his future with them.

2. Ben is still unable to verbalise his wishes and feelings regarding contact with his father easily, although he has made progress in stating to his social worker recently that he wished to cancel one of these visits. I remain concerned that Mr Jones may be unable to accommodate to Ben's growing assertiveness and independence from him, and may centre their contact sessions on activities which meet his own needs rather than those of Ben, as Mr Jones seemed to do following the above mentioned cancelled contact. Ideally, Ben will further develop his ability to articulate his wishes regarding contact with his father, who still seems emotionally important to Ben, although judging from his indirect communications in his play therapy sessions, currently in a very negative way. Close monitoring of Ben's wishes and feelings regarding his father, including his indirect communications, needs to continue, in my opinion. Weekly contacts already seem to be too frequent, both because of Ben's desire to immerse himself more fully in his new life and because the contacts themselves do not appear to be wholly positive for Ben. I would suggest fortnightly contacts in the immediate future, and close assessment of the effects of this change on both Ben and on his father.

3. I have no relevant information to put before the court from my work with Ben on his wishes and feelings regarding his mother, nor was this the stated purpose of my assessment. It does seem likely from my work, however, that this issue did not dominate his current emotional life; his relationship with his father, and his relationships in foster care and at school seem most important to him.

4. Because of the emotional damage Ben was likely to have sustained over a period of time with his father, and because his earlier relationship with his mother was disrupted suddenly, it is likely that Ben will have longer term therapeutic needs, even within a secure foster placement. He has shown in his assessment that he is able to utilise non-directive play therapy sessions and this seems a viable method for him in the near future. During his adolescence a counselling approach may be more suitable. Ben's foster carers may also need psychological help with difficult emotional issues connected to Ben's care. Ben will most likely find transitions in his own development (e.g. adolescence, independent adulthood and parenthood) more stressful emotionally than normal as well as any unexpected change of circumstances which may occur within his foster carers' family.

References from the body of the report were then given and it was signed, dated and sent to the instructing solicitor to file with the court.

PRACTICE ISSUES

Differences and similarities to sustained therapeutic work

Many of the practice considerations for play therapy assessments are the same as those for more sustained work: the setting, materials, the length of sessions and the arrangements for the time of the sessions in order to minimise disruption to the daily lives of the child and carers are similar to those described elsewhere in this book and in our earlier one. For assessments, as for sustained work, careful attention should be paid to the materials in the room, making materials available to the child which readily allow him or her to play out important past or current life events symbolically. For example, if a child is known to have undergone major surgery, a play hospital or doctor's bag seems called for. We are not advocating that the materials in the playroom be highly circumscribed, as in some direct interventions (see Wolff, 1986), and as in some techniques of play diagnosis and assessment used for clinical purposes described by Marvasti (1989). Any selection of materials which might suggest undue bias on the part of the therapist must also be avoided. (We discuss this issue, particularly in relation to the dangers of using anatomically correct dolls, in our earlier book.) The materials in non-directive work would offer a wide range of play opportunities, as illustrated in Ben's case, and remain the same each week. This continuity from one session to the next is important in both shorter and longer term work in order to assess changes within a child's functioning against a largely static background.

We examine significant similarities and differences between assessments and longer term therapy below, concentrating on writing court reports, appropriateness and timing of assessments, working with other professionals and issues of confidentiality.

Writing assessment reports for the court

Assessment reports are quite different from the brief reports the therapist submits to the statutory agency which are either kept in the confidential section of the child's file or given orally at case conferences. The latter reports would contain general statements of the child's therapeutic progress, and include only broad statements of concerns and issues which the child was addressing in the sessions. Assessment reports are more detailed; when a therapist writes such a report for the court, it is useful to keep the following points in mind.

First, the therapist needs continually to remain aware of the different audiences for whom the report is intended, as well as other readers who may have indirect access to it. Most importantly, the child may read a copy of the report during proceedings, if old enough, or may have other people relay some of the contents of the report. Even if the child has declined to read the report at the conclusion of the sessions he or she may hear about or read it later. The therapist has to be careful to word her report in such a way that the effect on the child will not be counter-therapeutic.

In Ben's case it was important that the therapist's report did not imply that Ben's aggression towards a father figure was at a dangerous, uncontrolled level or that Ben should be held responsible for his father's severe punishment of him. By setting out the positive aspects of Ben's personality and his progress in his sessions, the report attempts to create a sense of hopefulness in Ben himself should he have access to it at a later date. Other issues may not be as straightforward. For a child who maintains his emotional equilibrium by using the coping mechanism of blocking out all knowledge of his mother's rejection of him, as Ben may have done, having the therapist raise this issue and give it prominence in her report may be difficult for the child because he was not ready to address this issue. On the other hand, failing to mention this topic in the report would neglect a possibly important area of Ben's emotional life which might need later therapeutic intervention. The therapist had to give careful thought as to how to address this, in order to take account of

Ben's longer term needs as well as to give complete information to the court.

The therapist will have already assured both family and child that confidential material emerging in the child's sessions which is not directly relevant to proceedings will be respected and not included in her report. In a few cases, however, it may be difficult to decide whether to reveal information which has the potential to damage the family's ongoing relationship. Such material may leave the child open to blame and/or ridicule within the family, or may reveal new information to the child, such as, say, the true identity of his or her natural father. In these cases, while the therapist has the duty to report to the court all pertinent findings, she may alert the social worker for the family, the guardian, and the family itself about these 'family secrets' beforehand. In this way the family may have access to immediate professional help in dealing with these sensitive topics, before being involved in the court arena. The report should be written in a way which acknowledges sympathetically the painfulness for the family of involvement in court proceedings, and, because of their indirect effect on the child, may also consider the therapeutic needs of the adults in the case.

Another crucial audience for the therapist's report to the court are the legal representatives of the court, including the judge, barristers and solicitors for all parties. The main reason for requesting an expert's opinion in court proceedings is to provide the court with an experienced, objective view on a matter before the court. This has implications for the style and stance adopted in the report, and for the information it contains. As well as including all relevant information on the child, it should be jargon-free, written in a clear, unbiased and non-partisan style, and demonstrate an understanding of the distinction between fact, hypothesis and interpretation. In general ' . . . any contrary or inconsistent views [of other parties should be addressed] directly in the report . . . , providing a personal opinion on why they should not prevail over the expert's own views' (Gardner, 1994: 17). In Ben's report, for example, the therapist contrasted Ben's positive feelings about his current life in care with his negative feelings which were linked to his father, indicating that she considered his fearfulness to be due to his damaging earlier experiences rather than accepting alternative hypotheses that it resulted from being separated from his father or from unhappiness in his foster home.

The assessment report needs to stand on its own as a complete documentation of the expert's opinion for the court, since the therapist may not be called as a witness herself to give evidence and may not, therefore, be able to amplify points made in the document. There should be enough information in the report to establish the writer's credentials, by providing background details of her experience and professional qualifications, and a description of the method(s) of assessment used. The therapist should assume that any method used in assessment is liable to be scrutinized by the court, even if her method is accepted and practised inside her profession. With non-directive play therapy it is important to give a general statement to the court on the way in which this method of therapy is practised and the sessions recorded. In some court cases where other experts may be unfamiliar with this therapeutic method, the therapist may need to supplement her report by describing the history and tenets of this approach, as well as her safeguards to good practice, such as formulating working hypotheses and using information from sessional work and outside sources during the progress of sessions to evaluate and update her hypotheses.

In assessment reports, similarly to reports of therapeutic work for the court, the therapist will give primacy to her direct work with the child. It is also important, however, that her other sources of information are precisely documented, with dates, and can be seen by the court to be thorough. It may be prudent to explain the reasons for not seeing a parent or another party who might arguably be significant to the child, such as Ben's mother. In working with a guardian, as in Ben's case, the therapist will assume that the guardian is responsible for thorough coverage of the child's history, including all information in the social services file. However, the therapist may decide that in order to form her opinion, she requires more information than is given to her in her meeting with the guardian and social services' personnel. In Ben's case, for example, she asked for the case notes on file regarding supervised contact visits with his father.

It is relatively more important to include these outside sources of information in court assessments of the child, than in reports to the court of longer term therapeutic work with a child. In longer term work the therapist needs a working knowledge of the child's life in order to understand the child's ongoing thoughts and feelings more easily, and, of course, always needs information in order to be alert to ongoing child protection issues which may arise during their sessions. In contrast, the period for an assessment is briefer, the therapist will probably not be as familiar with the child's world as she would be in a longer term therapeutic relationship, and outside sources may provide needed information on areas which are not spontaneously covered by the child in play sessions. The therapist also uses information derived from other sources to supplement and compare with information from the child's play and verbal communications during sessions. Thus, the therapist used the information which the teacher had provided to the social worker about Ben's night in the shed, for instance, in order to follow his play communication more accurately and in order to inform her opinion on Ben's allegation of abuse by his father.

It should be stressed, however, that the therapist's opinion of possible abuse of Ben by his father was not based only on a particular play sequence, even if it was a very powerful one, from Ben's play sessions. Information derived from all his sessions by the therapist needed to coalesce and form a coherent set of hypotheses, as we explain more fully below. Equally importantly, the information from the child's sessions must be weighed against all the other sources of information to which the therapist has access, in order to conduct a multidimensional, thorough assessment of the child.

As well as outside sources, it is assumed that the therapist as an expert will draw on and cite selective research and theory in her field, in this case the relevant child development, child abuse and child therapy literatures. These should be familiar to the other child care professionals involved and, although legal professionals may not know specific references, they will be trained in legal aspects related to child abuse and child development and will be generally familiar with concepts, and some of the literature in these areas. With Ben's report, for instance, the therapist thought it important to refer to the patterns of expected responses described in the psychological literature for children recovering from trauma.

The final important audience which the therapist addresses in the report is the local authority, who will be legally responsible for the child under all court orders. By providing an outside psychological opinion based upon direct work with the child, the therapist is able to offer another perspective to social workers and their legal representatives in meeting a child's needs, especially in the kinds of cases for which a therapeutic assessment seems warranted. When the therapist is instructed by the local authority rather than the guardian, her role remains unchanged. She is not an advocate for the local authority's position; the therapist continues to assess the case for the *child's* best interests and provide an expert opinion for the court. In our experience the therapist can be helpful to local authority professionals in their formulation of a care plan for the child at earlier stages in the proceedings. Her report also can help to focus their attention on key issues for the child in complex cases. With local authority funding constraints and allocation of resources a constant factor in care decisions, the report can also be useful in the 'Recommendations' section by giving guidance on realistic shorter term and longer term needs of the child. With Ben, for example, the therapist endorsed the local authority's care plan for him, as well as specifying his later therapeutic needs and a possible change of contact arrangements with his father. While the therapist does not need to have special knowledge of the ways in which these recommendations should be turned into legally binding agreements, as the guardian, social worker and legal representatives of the parties do, it is useful for her to have a working knowledge of how orders can be specified by the court and the ways in which social services intend to implement them.

We consider finally in this section the key question of how the evidence derived from play therapy sessions should be presented. As we have seen, Ben's report began with a general description of his personality, derived from the therapist's observations of him and knowledge of normal and abused children, followed by an account of the changes manifested over the period of the assessment. A factual description of the contents of the sessions together was then given. Since the report is a summary, rather than a detailed account of each session, we advocate that the therapist study the contents of the sessions and draw out key emotional themes for the child. During this analytical process all the examples from each session are, as befits descriptive data, 'compared to each other in order first to generate and then to confirm, refine and relate emergent categories' (Giffin, 1984: 78). These catogories, or themes are generated from the examples themselves, and from the therapist's knowledge and experience of children's emotional, social, cognitive and physical development.

This task is made easier, as we saw in Ben's case, because troubled children often have a limited number of intensely important personal themes which are identifiable in their sessions. Ben's theme of fearfulness was derived first from Ben himself and then related to the therapist's knowledge of children's emotional development. In very young children, who are beginning to increase their autonomy and independence from adult carers, the therapist would have thought it normal to have seen some play around monsters and fear of outside attack. In boys in middle childhood, the therapist would also have thought it normal that aggression and fear of personal safety from outside agents was present in their play. However, with Ben the intensity of his fear in his play with monsters was more extreme than normal. His later sessions then showed an intense fear related to a father figure, which again exceeded normal limits. (We will discuss further in the next section on theoretical issues the ways in which fantasy and reality contributed to Ben's play themes.)

Sometimes the therapist may have difficulty in picking out relevant themes, especially in sessions which are highly complex ones with many interrelating emotional issues for the child. The task is often made more demanding when longer term therapy has been conducted with the child, than in shorter term therapy for court assessments. There will be a greater amount of sessional material as well as changes in focus, which the child may instigate as therapy progresses. In both types of work, however, the therapist may have to think carefully about differing explanations and about the child's use of different metaphors and symbolic expressions for the same underlying theme (Siegelman, 1990). As Moore discusses with children's drawings, and as we have stated in our earlier book, symbolic representations allow 'many levels of self-experience to be accessed and depicted simultaneously' (1994a: 225). Some of these meanings, as we discuss below, may be inaccessible to the therapist. She may have to keep an open mind, and decide that she is unable to relate particular play behaviours to any of her main themes or any other known issues in the child's life with any high degree of probability.

Certain themes discussed by the therapist in her report on a child's play therapy sessions will arise from the instructions from the acting solicitor which were received by the therapist. In many cases these instructions correlate well with the issues raised by the child in his play sessions. However, at times issues relevant for the court assessment are absent from the child's sessions. In these cases, the therapist has to think carefully in the light of other information derived both from the child's sessions and other sources about possible reasons for this omission. For example, a child such as Ben, who knows that his sessions are about his relationship with his father, but who makes no mention of a father figure or male role in his direct communications, or his play material in any of his six sessions, may have a variety of reasons for this omission. The therapist would have to give her opinion on the possible reason(s) for this in her report, such as a lack of interest in his father, an unusual fear of this topic, or a failure to trust the therapist, to name just a few possibilities.

In summary, the therapist, in writing her assessment report for the court, should attempt to present facts, hypotheses and opinions in a clear, succinct and objective manner in order to aid the court's decisions regarding what is best for a particular child.

The appropriateness and timing of therapeutic assessments

In this section we consider through Ben's story the way in which play therapy can be used as a method of assessment of the child's developmental needs, wishes and feelings in statutory proceedings. This method of assessment has evolved from the first author's presentation in court of evidence derived from longer term play therapy work with children (see Wilson et al., 1992: Chapter 7). It is assumed with this type of assessment that a child's individual needs, wishes and feelings can be identified by forming a therapeutic relationship with him or her. For this reason the assessment is carried out over approximately a six-week period, involving weekly sessions with the child. This method of assessment, using non-directive play therapy, also seems to be highly responsive to recent legal changes in British courts.

We have indicated in our earlier discussion some of the ways in which play therapy for assessment purposes differs from longer term work with children. It is (usually) briefer, and this clearly may have an impact on the child's ability to explore core concerns. (See Diane for an illustration of changes in therapy following the funding of further sessions.) The therapist may make more use of outside sources because of her relative lack of familiarity with the child's environment. The limited confidentiality which the therapist can offer, due to the need to report to the courts, may restrict the child's level of engagement in therapy. This may be particularly the case with older children, who have a greater understanding of the implications of court hearings, whereas other children may be relatively unconcerned.

Yet other children appear to engage deeply in sessions because play enactments are their preferred way of conveying their needs, wishes and feelings to the court and do not seem strongly to differ from children in longer term work. As we saw with Ben, the sessions allow the child to explore important personal themes to therapeutic effect. Indeed, an advantage when non-directive play therapy is used for court assessment purposes is that a short series of non-directive play therapy sessions is in this way automatically made available to the child. (Family and child psychiatrists and family therapists, as well as therapists with individual assessments, may also use a therapeutic approach in their work for the courts.) Not only, as we saw with Ben, will these short-term therapeutic sessions potentially be of benefit to the child immediately, it is also a way in which the child's longer term therapeutic needs can be recognised, and be more likely to be acted upon by the local authority and health services.

Such assessments by an outside professional may be asked for in a range of circumstances. New requirements were put upon British courts with the implementation of the Children Act 1989. Since that date the courts have a duty placed on them to ascertain the child's wishes, feelings and developmental needs in any course of action in which a child is directly involved, in an effort to protect a child's needs from being subordinated to those of adults. A guardian *ad litem* is appointed to represent the child's interests for the duration of court proceedings, giving the child a voice and a professional who is independent from both family members and from the statutory agency involved. It is intended, and is normally the case, that the guardian is the professional who works directly with the child, helping the child communicate verbally, often with the use of play materials to facilitate this process, his or her wishes, feelings and needs concerning the matter before the court. In some cases, however, the guardian may apply to the court for an outside professional assessment. Reasons for this assessment can include children who have difficulties in direct communication. Among these children may be those who are too young, too frightened or too inhibited to state their wishes and feelings directly. Others may have severe emotional conflicts or emotional confusion over issues before the court, and indirect psychological methods may be preferable in order to minimise the possibility of retraumatisation by a professional. At other times the issues for the child are complex, and an independent psychological or psychiatric opinion is asked for in order to clarify the child's current and future developmental needs, including therapeutic needs. Finally, some cases are more contentious and would benefit from the expertise of a professional opinion.

Statutory agencies have similar reasons for asking for independent assessments. The case may be complex and/or the child may have difficulty articulating his own needs, wishes and feelings to his social worker. In addition, the social worker for the child may be the worker for the entire sibling group in the family and be directly involved in working with the parents, extended family or carers of the child. With complex family issues or with conflicts of interests among siblings or among the children and parents, an independent assessment may be sought. Given budgetary constraints in statutory agencies, in practice it is most often in contested, or potentially contested, cases that an independent view is sought, with the intent that this view will inform opinions and avoid or lessen controversy in court, while maintaining the focus of all parties on the child's interests.

Direct methods of arriving at the child's needs, wishes and feelings for the court may, then, either be unworkable or need further amplification. In these circumstances, evidence derived from non-directive play therapy may be a valuable source of information as to the child's state of mind. Non-directive play therapy, as we have seen in Ben's sessions, is an important means of arriving indirectly at both a child's current state of mind and his developmental needs. In addition, it seems particularly well adapted to court purposes, since it is child-centred, non-coercive and largely free from interpretation and suggestion (Wilson et al., 1992; Ryan and Wilson, 1995b).

In addition to the court's enhanced requirements of evidence related to the child's wishes and feelings, embodied in the Children Act 1989, concern about the quality of evidence for court proceedings involving children has been reflected in two major documents, namely the Criminal Justice Act 1991 and the Memorandum of Good Practice 1992. In the former, recognition of the difficulties arising from restrictions in the testimony of child witnesses to abuse who were the only witness to the alleged offence, led to new provisions for child witnesses. In the latter, criticisms of investigative interviews of children which were unduly suggestive and leading have resulted in changes in interviewing techniques. These developments make it vital that communications which may be used for evidential purposes are non-coercive, avoid using leading questions and show an open-mindedness about the occurrence and meaning of events. As we argue elsewhere, key features of non-directive play therapy are well adapted to these requirements, for the following reasons (Ryan and Wilson, 1995b: 160):

1. The child chooses the activities or themes in the session; the suggestive effects which might be adduced if the therapist selected the focus of the session are minimised.
2. The permissive atmosphere encourages the child to choose and explore themes which are meaningful and of concern to him. Evidence of play therapy themes thus is likely to reflect the child's real preoccupations.
3. The accuracy of reports from play therapy sessions is enhanced because the permissive atmosphere encourages the child to correct, reject or ignore any response from the therapist which, for whatever reason, does not 'fit' with his current concern.
4. The therapist's response to the child's activity is one of reflection rather than interpretation. Thus the likelihood that the child's further explorations, verbally or non-verbally, arise as a result of suggestions on the part of the therapist as to the primacy, aetiology or cause of a particular activity or concern is minimised.

As we have shown, the therapist in her sessions with Ben was open to his view of the occurrence of events and to the events which he identified as being emotionally important to him. She avoided the use of leading questions and suggestion. For example, when Ben drew the man with holes in him during the first session, she did not ask him whether that man was his dad or someone else. She made a tentative, non-threatening remark that perhaps something was wrong with the man, which Ben would hopefully have been able to correct, reject or ignore if he did not wish to pursue this activity. In this sense, it should be clarified, the therapist's role in non-directive play therapy *is* therapeutically suggestive, but only in a highly circumscribed way. Her reflection of what Ben was feeling and expressing, and her manner was based on her own understanding of his inner world. Of course, if therapy is to be effective for a child, it is assumed that the therapist's accurate reflections *will* have some influence on the child's subsequent actions, thoughts and feelings. In Ben's case he then chose to develop this activity in his own manner, becoming more overtly aggressive and pretending to shoot bullet holes into this cartoon man, killing him and finally 'rubbing him out' (both literally and metaphorically).

The therapist would not have altered her response and become more directive and leading, either when undertaking longer term work or when the evidence was needed for the court. Ben would easily in her opinion have become too threatened emotionally at this stage in their sessions together and might have erected greater emotional defences against this topic as a result. Suggestion of the contents to be explored in their sessions, such as asking Ben to play out what he felt about his dad, or therapeutic interpretations, such as 'you must have suffered badly with that man to want to shoot and kill him like that' might well have hindered the purpose of their non-directive play therapy sessions together, which is to encourage the *child* to choose the material to be explored and to arrive at *his own* understanding of it (Ryan and Wilson, 1995b). (See also p. 225 onwards in this chapter for a discussion of more subtle forms of bias and unintentional suggestion by the therapist.)

Restrictions on conducting therapeutic assessments

We should make clear, however, that in a few cases an assessment of a child using non-directive play therapy may be detrimental to the child's welfare. (These considerations are similar to those discussed in Susan's case, chapter 1, for longer term play therapy.) Some assessments should more properly be conducted by a psychiatrist or another specialist, given the known background of the child or the family. In certain cases the evidence may be medical, rather than psychological, and a paediatrician may be the professional who will more properly conduct the assessment and offer a professional opinion to the court. In other cases it may be that the therapist's opinion based on referral information is that the child is already unsafe in his or her current environment, and would be at even greater risk of abuse if play-therapy sessions were to start. In these cases the therapist may request to the court that the child be removed to and settled into a safer environment prior to her commencing work with the child, giving her reasons for doing so. These reasons would include indicators of significant risk of harm to the child, such as some cases of disclosure of abuse by the child, the sustaining of serious injuries or harm already by the child, or the lack of demonstration by the carer that the child is protected in a risk situation.

At other times the child may not be adequately supported for this type of therapeutic assessment by his or her placement. It may be that the therapist is asked to step in to do an assessment at an early stage in a statutory agency's work with parents or other carers of the child. Legal proceedings may not be sought immediately because, in the local authority's judgement, the child does not seem at immediate risk of harm in his or her current environment. In these cases the therapist will have to make a judgement herself on whether the carers are sufficiently motivated to bring the child to play therapy sessions and whether the intervention itself will contribute to a higher risk situation for the child. It may not be of value to the child to embark on a number of play sessions, and then not be allowed to continue these sessions if the carers decide otherwise or fail to keep appointments. The statutory agency and therefore the therapist herself will be dependent on the voluntary agreement of the child's carers to the assessment itself, and to the therapist's use of video or audiorecordings. In some circumstances the children may be accommodated by the local authority with the parents' or carers' agreement. They will then have the right to withhold their consent for the type of intervention which they allow professionals to conduct with their child.

In all cases in which the parents are emotionally involved with the child, regardless of their legal rights, it is important that the therapist tries to introduce herself to the child's parents and attempts to persuade them that the type of intervention she is conducting will serve the needs of their child. The child's parents will often rightly be concerned that the therapist, a stranger to them, will see their child and may, through insensitive intervention, harm their child emotionally (This lack of complete trust in child care professionals is warranted by parents, as certain cases of overzealous or abusive therapeutic and social work interventions demonstrate.) Meeting the therapist is a direct way in which the parents may be able to relieve their anxiety for their child and have the opportunity to ask the therapist questions which concern them.

The non-directive method is in itself readily understandable by parents as being non-intrusive and, because it is set in a play context, it will usually reassure them that it is less likely to increase their child's anxiety that more direct methods. The method itself also is readily understood by parents as being non-suggestive and sensitive to the child's wishes and feelings. The therapist is able to assure the child's parents that she will not ask questions of the child, nor will she be partisan in any disputes that may have arisen for the parents with any other agencies, professionals, or other interested parties, such as grandparents or an estranged partner. Similarly to the therapist's position with the child and with the court, the therapist tries to encourage the parents to view her as solely representing the child's interests, and not on one or the other side of an adversarial dispute.

The therapist is in a prime position to focus parents on issues that are of urgency for their child and can be a catalyst for positive change in the child's parents, if her interview with them is conducted with an attitude of helpfulness to a troubled family, rather than in a confrontational manner (see chapter 4). The therapist may decide in some cases to wait a few weeks until her assessment is under way to introduce herself to the child's parents, as in Ben's case, where the parents do not have the day-to-day care of the child or the child's legal care. This short delay may be necessary to keep the cost of the assessment within reasonable boundaries, making one interview with the parents suffice. The therapist's role in an assessment, unlike longer term therapy, would be more limited with carers and parents. The social worker would be responsible for this aspect of work in the case. The therapist may, therefore, decide that after she has started working with the child, she will then be in a better position to identify clearly issues to discuss with the parents from the child's point of view. In all cases where the parents have the day-to-day care of the child without legal proceedings under way, it remains very important that the therapist interview the parents prior to working with the child to assess whether this type of intervention is appropriate as well as to enlist their close cooperation, in addition to meeting them during her intervention.

In cases where the child is accommodated by the local authority, a play-therapy assessment may in a few cases still not be feasible because of other competing demands on the foster carer's time. In these cases, as in longer term therapeutic work, there should be a thorough examination of whether these overstretched circumstances are temporary or whether the placement generally is inadequate for the child's needs. Rarely, in our experience, is the assessment not supported by either the child's foster carers or the child's social worker. On the very few occasions in which a lack of social work support has occurred in our practice, either the social worker herself or himself wished to conduct the work or judged that no therapeutic intervention was needed.

Sometimes the child is to move placements shortly, and this issue is most properly of dominant concern both to him and to adults. There may not be enough investment by carers, the child, or professionals, because of this major upheaval, for the child to benefit from therapeutic work. Generally it must be recognised that a therapeutic assessment as we have detailed here *does* require more effort and commitment on the part of the child's carer and social worker, the former having to allocate time to bring the child to his sessions and the latter often becoming involved in transport arrangements and funding requests. The child's environment is also crucial in promoting and stabilising therapeutic changes in the child. The carers and social workers would be working in partnership with the therapist in a close manner in a therapeutic assessment, as we detailed in our earlier chapters on longer term work.

Another consideration in deciding whether a play therapy assessment is of value to the child is when a child has several professional or parent/carer relationships already. Another relationship with a new adult may create confusion in the child or may hamper him from forming closer attachments to appropriate adults in his life. We have stated in our earlier book that the therapist should not be in the position of being the child's main attachment figure, which would be a misuse of the therapeutic relationship. (In longer term therapeutic work it may be more appropriate in cases where the child has a previous history of broken or diffuse attachments for the play therapist to consider supervising a professional carer, or consulting with another professional the child is already engaged within therapeutic work. However, the obvious disadvantage of consultations if the child is involved in court proceedings is that the therapist's evidence would not then be based on direct knowledge of the child himself and may therefore weaken her opinions in court.)

Once a therapeutic assessment is completed, a child or young person should have the option of continuing with play-therapy sessions, if the child so wishes and if the therapist agrees that this is the appropriate intervention for the child. This change from shorter to longer term work would be treated by the therapist as similar to coming to the end of a set of agreed sessions in longer term work, and assessing, in consultation with relevant others, whether the child will continue. [See discussion in Wilson et al. (1992: chapter 3) on the advantages of time-limited interventions in longer term work.]

Finally, if a therapeutic assessment would in any way unnecessarily delay court proceedings for the child, and therefore add further because of this to the environmental and emotional instability in his life, a shorter type of assessment, such as psychological testing within a clinical interview, may be preferred. While this type of assessment would give the court a different kind of information, since the assessment would be adult-led, and would not usually involve seeing the child over a period of time and establishing a therapeutic relationship, it may be the preferred method of assessment when other constraints exist.

The overall potential benefits and disadvantages to the child of a court assessment based on non-directive play therapy must therefore be weighed up carefully before embarking on this type of assessment.

Other methods of psychological assessment

Certain types of psychological testing will have the advantage of objectively developed reliability and validity scales, unlike therapeutic assessments which are based upon the therapist's professional clinical opinion. Relevant information for assessment purposes may be elicited from the child more quickly and efficiently, and will be able to be replicated by others. However, with children who are not able to easily impart information directly to professionals, either because of their inherent limitations, such as age, cognitive and language capacities, or because of their emotional difficulties, psychological testing and/or interviewing may have several disadvantages. First, direct questioning or probing, as well as being suggestive, may also be experienced by the child as intrusive and anxiety-provoking. In more seriously abused and traumatised children, these methods could run the risk of retraumatising the child (Moore, 1995). Second, questions which allow open-ended recall of information by a child who has these kinds of individual limitations often provide only minimal information (Spencer and Flin, 1990). Third, when direct methods are employed, the child may not have access to traumatic memories on a conscious, verbal level and therefore may not provide the court with the same kind of information as that derived from either a play-therapy assessment or from an interview using projective techniques (Ryan and Wilson, 1995b).

Projective tests have the advantage of not relying on direct questioning of the child, yet some lack sound reliability and validity scales, and thus may be limited to giving useful pointers in arriving at a clinical opinion. Other tests, such as the human figure drawings test, will have more validity and reliability because they are based on normative, cross-cultural data (Moore, 1994b). However, no projective data, as Moore cautions in regard to drawings, owing to the subjective nature of the projective and interpretive processes involved in any projective technique, should be utilised on their own for alleging abuse or assigning a diagnostic label, but should be 'correlated with other independent sources of information in a multi-dimensional assessment of a child' (1994a: 221), a view we have already expressed when using play material for court purposes.

Certain projective techniques with children, for example, the Bene-Anthony Family Relations Test with supplementary cards, have been developed for assessing potentially abusive situations. This test has recently been advocated as providing the child with an inbuilt structure during assessment interviews while remaining non-directive (Mertin and Rooney, 1995). However, the test does not reliably differentiate clinical from non-clinical populations, partly because of the wide range of individual responses which a child can make to the test materials. While the cards do provide the child with a relatively non-threatening, age-appropriate structure within which to talk about their experiences, the topics in the test materials do seem to be suggestive (e.g. 'This person touches my bottom'). They are 'non-directive', as the authors claim, only in the sense that they are *less* directive than specific questions and do not assign an adult value judgement to any statement. They remain directive because the adult still determines the concerns which the child addresses. (Another potential concern is that the category of 'Mr Nobody' to which the child can assign any of the cards may not be a sufficient safeguard to counteract the effect of the interviewer's position of authority in possibly eliciting an unknown or a compliant response in a child.)

The above test and others, such as the House-Tree-Person Test, the Kinetic Family Drawing Test, the Blacky Test or the Three Wishes Test, while not psychologically reliable and valid, still can be clinically useful for the therapist in suggesting interpretations regarding the child's self-concept, themes which are emotionally important to the child and his or her possible defences against emotionally difficult experiences. These tests, of course, can also be used by the therapist in ongoing therapeutic assessments and longer term non-directive play therapy with a child, as we discussed in our earlier book, by incorporating structured exercises into a non-directive approach. Singer (1993) also illustrates uses of projective tests and guided imagery in her case presentations.

Confidentiality and recording in court assessments

There are different views concerning the need for complete recordings of therapeutic sessions for court-related work. Some therapists advocate that all interactions with the child be recorded in order to stand on their own. When the sessions are with child witnesses to criminal proceedings, the court may make machine recording of sessions a requirement in order to allow work to be done with the child prior to proceedings while simultaneously guarding against contamination of the child's evidence. Care proceedings and contact applications can also be highly contentious. The court may order that the therapist's records be turned over to another expert's opinion or to other parties in the proceedings. If the therapist has tapes which were transcribed by her after each session and on which she bases her examples and opinions in her court report, they can be used as evidence along with her case notes. Her recordings can then be scrutinised in detail for the presence or absence of bias, suggestion and leading questions by counsel. Recordings can also be an added safeguard for the therapist who is alone in the playroom with the child, if the child were to make an allegation against the therapist regarding physical, emotional or sexual abuse.

Recording sessions is also a check on the therapist's memory for events, and is a necessity in our opinion if the sessions are not written up in full immediately after a session or if the action or dialogue was confusing to follow or very rapid. This practice seems especially important when the therapist works alone, without an observer present to verify and check on the therapist's practice. While some therapists rely on an observer behind a one-way screen to correct for therapist bias and to provide an accurate recording of events during sessions, perhaps along with machine recordings, we consider generally that machine recordings alone of the sessions with the child are less intrusive. The child does not have to take into account other people's opinions of his or her actions, nor do they have such a public quality. (Although even with recording equipment, the child may 'play to' the camera and adopt a more public persona, or become overly inhibited because of its intrusiveness.)

If the sessions are adequately documented by using recordings of the sessions, and if the therapist does not spend additional, undocumented time with the child outside of their sessions together, the therapist will be able to give an undertaking to the court that leading questions, unwarranted suggestion and interpretation have not been used, and thus have not contaminated the child's evidence during their sessions, nor has she conducted a biased assessment. Recordings of sessions, then, can be seen as safeguards for the child, the court and the therapist that the therapist is representing information from her assessment accurately and fully.

There are, however, some difficulties with full recordings being used for court purposes. First of all, the child may object to the intrusion of the recordings. In these cases, as we stated earlier (Wilson et al., 1992), the therapist can argue this difficulty before the court, if the court has required this documentation, as not being in the best interests of the child. Second, it is misleading to assume that even complete video recordings will give full information to other professionals who were not present at the actual event itself. Research into investigative interviewing methods using video (e.g. Westcott et al., 1991) and studies on emotional expression (Ekman et al., 1980) have indicated that a child's and an adult's emotional expressions rely on subtle changes of facial expression, voice tone and small motor movements (Heard and Lake's (1986) 'emotive messages'). Because of the multiple indicators of emotions relied on in direct communication, a video recording will attenuate the strength as well as the subtlety of the participants' emotional expressions. Furthermore, in order to circumvent this problem at least partially, strict guidelines for full-face video recordings are specified in investigative interviews used for evidential purposes. These guidelines, however, are unsuitable for play therapy sessions because of their severe restrictions on the child's movements, among other reasons. (See the Home Office (1992) Memorandum of Good Practice.)

The court will already have needed to give permission for an assessment (or therapeutic work) to be conducted prior to play therapy sessions starting. Following recent court practice, the therapist should assume that all her clinical material, including notes, tapes and letters can be called as evidence in civil or criminal proceedings. These will be subject potentially to scrutiny by the court, including the judge and all parties' legal representatives. This may or may not include the parties to the proceedings. Other experts called upon to advise in the case may also be asked to examine these papers (Jakobi and Pratt, 1992; Tufnell, 1995). It will be difficult for legal representatives and other parties to the proceedings, as well as other experts who are not child psychologists or play therapists themselves, or who are unpractised in a non-directive approach, to be knowledgeable about the meaning of the contents of non-directive play-therapy sessions with the child.

Even very basic details in the contents of the child's therapy sessions may be misleading to non-experts. The therapist herself may also unwittingly convey suggestions to the child very subtly and outside her conscious knowledge, for example, through the use of more highly emotive words for emotions which are in fact more weakly expressed by the child (e.g. 'cross', 'a bit angry' or *very* angry'). The therapist's actions can also convey information to the child about her attitudes to him that are not readily apparent in recordings, for example, with an intense stare the therapist may unduly call the child's attention to the doll's genitals as the child takes off the doll's clothes, having not attended initially himself to that area of the doll's body. On the other hand, the therapist may be indifferent to what the child has demonstrated an interest in. The integrity of the therapist and her access to supervision of her cases as a protection against her personal attitudes and prejudices, then, may be an important issue at the outset of precourt discussions. While precourt discussions with experts may eliminate some of these differences in interpretation of the material from sessions, or show bias in the therapist, very detailed scrutiny of the sessions and point by point discussions may often be necessary in order to establish valid differences of opinion between experts.

It also seems in children's best interests to keep their personal information from sessions as private and confidential as possible, even within a court setting. Children are usually too young to give informed consent and it would then be the therapist's role to protect their privacy and to foresee possible consequences, both shorter term and longer term, from disclosure of private material. The therapist may ask the judge in the case first of all to refuse permission for release of her papers to safeguard the child's privacy. If the judge rules that, in the interests of justice, information must be made available to the other parties in the case or to another expert, the therapist may ask the judge for a ruling that the court keep a single copy of the materials on file at court for perusal, rather than having the materials duplicated and distributed to other parties' counsel, with the risks of the material not being secure or not being shredded or returned after use to the therapist. While there is a growing practice of experts returning materials to source after proceedings, safeguards to the strict confidentiality of materials and return of documents is not to date well established in law (personal communication, Mrs D. Adcock, 1995). Safeguarding of confidential documents is an issue for any agency or private practitioner.

This feature of therapeutic work in a court setting has obvious implications for the confidentiality which can be offered to the child by the therapist and to any of the parties involved with the child. The limit to confidentiality is very apparent, and the therapist needs to make it clear that, although she will do as much as she can to respect confidences, anything that is relevant to a decision concerning a child or to criminal proceedings is within the jurisdiction of the court and may need to be divulged. (We discuss the impact that this may have on therapy more fully in Patricia's chapter.)

Working with other professionals

We have already discussed the therapist's need to work in partnership with other professionals in longer term therapeutic work with a child (see chapter 1, Susan; Ryan, 1994; Wilson and Ryan, 1994b). As Ben's story illustrates, the therapist conducting an assessment for the court also needs to work closely with other professionals involved in the legal proceedings. We have already seen that the guardian represents the child's interests in any proceedings directly affecting a child, and he or she would be one of the key professionals with whom the therapist would work. The guardian's role, helped by his solicitor, would also be to coordinate precourt meetings of two or more experts where necessary, to try to reach agreement among experts, particularly those of the same discipline. This practice is intended to eliminate the use of court time in expert disputes by having experts agree on as many as possible of the contentious issues in the case prior to the hearing itself (Trett, 1994). It also has the advantage of serving to remove expert discussions from an adversarial setting. There has recently been a proposition in the case of Re G by Mr Justice Wall (1994) that, in children's cases, an attempt should be made to limit in any given category of evidence the number of experts in the same discipline who will be instructed by the court (Tufnell, 1995).

Following from this judicial opinion it seems that an expert in child cases is increasingly being recognised as an expert 'for the court' (Gardner, 1994). This shift in legal practice means that British child cases are more closely modelled on the role of the expert in non-adversarial legal systems in which a court-appointed expert informs judicial decisions, such as that of the German criminal justice system (Terheyden, 1995). The judge in a children's case, then, may not grant leave for multiple appointments of experts in a given category of evidence, e.g. two child and family psychiatrists to examine the child independently (Tufnell, 1995). This practice has the additional advantage for the child that he is not subjected to any more professional intrusion than is necessary for an expert to form an opinion.

In general with assessments of the child for the court, the therapist needs to be informed of the opinions of the other experts and of other developments in the case which will affect her own opinion. In Ben's case, the professionals were in agreement, where their opinions were available, concerning his father's attitudes and behaviour. In other cases, however, professionals' opinions may not concur or the information at their disposal may not be sufficient from other sources to form an opinion. Another expert's assessment may then be much more crucial. Even within the same field, professionals' methods, training and theoretical background may differ. Open-mindedness to other viewpoints is needed and sometimes difficult to achieve. Also, these 'differences of opinion' can mask wider issues of professional jealousy, genuine worries about professional incompetence, the inadvertent mirroring of a dysfunctional family system by the professional system, and at times a failure to focus on the child's needs. Often it is obvious that there are heightened needs of adult parties in the proceedings, which other professionals may be assessing and which may mask or attenuate a focus on the child. For these reasons and for wider general use by the court, it is important that the expert use non-technical language where possible and explain their methods clearly. The expert should also be thorough in reporting on findings, have a willingness to admit areas of information not yet available for consideration and a willingness to incorporate other professionals' viewpoints into his or her own opinion.

This level of objectivity is, we have argued elsewhere (Ryan and Wilson, 1995b) much easier for the therapist to state in the abstract than it is to sustain in practice. The therapist will have had to adopt an empathic attitude towards the child in order to develop a working relationship with him. Also, as is evident with Ben, therapeutic material often has a high emotional content. Both these attributes may contribute to the therapist tending to give inordinate weight in court proceedings to information derived from her sessions with the child, and to devaluing evidence available from outside sources. Therefore, because of her personal relationship with the child, the therapist will have to make a more strenuous effort to maintain her objectivity. She will need to supplement her own awareness of possible bias with support from her supervisor/consultant. Similarly to our earlier argument that the practice of non-directive therapy entails the forming of hypotheses and weighing of alternatives, and therefore has already engendered skills in the therapist which are needed in court work, we would again stress that a tendency of the therapist to overidentify with the child is neither conducive to sound therapeutic practice *nor* to sound court practice.

Finally, the therapist will have to struggle with the knowledge that her work with the child will be open to close scrutiny for bias and suggestion by professionals who are not trained in therapeutic work themselves, and perhaps not sympathetic to her account. The therapist may become inhibited and passive in her work with the child in a misguided attempt to counteract potential criticism during court proceedings of undue suggestion and bias. Through support in supervision, careful use of non-directive skills during sessions and examination of the transcripts of sessions with the child, the therapist herself should 'be aware of places in sessions in which her minimal suggestions were necessary therapeutically because they were based on the child's behaviours. Since her concern above all is for the well-being of the child she must equally however, not be overly constrained by court proceedings, so that she is still able to use these suggestions in her reflections of the child's feelings effectively' (Ryan and Wilson, 1995b: 171).

THEORETICAL ISSUE

Distinguishing the child's wishes, feelings and fantasies from real current and past life events

As we have seen in this chapter, using play therapy material for court assessments is a complex, multi-faceted undertaking. With children who have had potentially traumatic or difficult life experiences which also will always interact with their innate constitutional disposition, a diagnostic label or definitive assessment for the court may be potentially misleading and unhelpful. A clearer picture of a complex problem is often gained only by sustained work with the child, noting how he or she responds to an enriched and individualised environment which attempts to redress earlier possible deficits and/or abuse. [See, for example, the detailed account of 'Marty' in Singer (1993).] Young children, in addition to any changes in their environments, often change their intellectual and emotional behaviour unpredictably in a relatively short time because of their rapid development.

We have also argued in this chapter that a non-directive play therapy assessment circumvents many of the problems raised in child witness research, which shows that children, especially those who are young and/

or who are in environments where they perceive adults as more knowing and more powerful, are then more vulnerable either to adult coercion and suggestion or to remaining silent (Spencer and Flin, 1990). By providing a permissive play environment in which the adult's role is that of a facilitator of the child's communications, rather that a director of them, the child is then largely free of the effects of suggestion and coercion. However, because the child's communications are often largely within a play metaphor, as Ben illustrates, a crucial issue is how the therapist can then assess whether the child's play is reality- or fantasy-based. We have seen that this consideration is to some extent part of any therapeutic work and is of central importance when, as with Patrick, he was making an allegation of abuse by his parents. The therapist needed to remain non-directive, and yet had to clarify the statements that Patrick made without curtailing or changing the substance of his remarks.

In situations in which the child is alleging abuse within his current environment, this clarification is of heightened urgency and the therapist must make a judgement as to whether or not to notify the child protection agency immediately. Both the child's verbal statements and his non-verbal behaviours may need clarifications which remain non-suggestive, as we discussed in an earlier chapter regarding Patrick's allegation of past abuse during a session. (See also Wilson et al., 1992.) The therapist, in completing her assessment for the court, would fully analyse this pertinent information from the child along with all the other information from within her sessions and from independent sources in order to offer an opinion on whether the child was making an accurate statement of abuse. Considerations of possible motives for truth or falsehood based on the child's choice of words, his or her description of the events themselves, the non-verbal components of the statement, the child's personality and defence mechanisms, would be undertaken, which are ultimately based on firm theoretical and research underpinnings, in a manner similar to the analysis of statements derived from investigative interviews (Raskin and Esplin, 1991).

Often, however, as Ben's story illustrates, the child's play communications are more complex, interweaving what appear to be elements of reality with fantasy. Some of the same criteria for analysis of play communications would apply which we have mentioned above with statement validity analysis. Analysing, for example, a child's language usage within his play productions, the therapist would ask herself questions such as: is the child's language of the same complexity as his or her ordinary productions? If not, is there an explanation based on the incident depicted? That is, does a boy of ten employ four-year-old language because the incident he is portraying occurred for him at four years of age? Has the child regressed to an earlier level of functioning because the content has a high emotional content which precludes his usual use of cognitive skills? Or is the language stilted because the child seems to be either fabricating the incident or mimicking an older person's vocabulary? Is it possible in this case that the child was coached or given suggestions by an adult or has overheard an emotionally charged scene between adults and is playing out these experiences? Has the child been exposed to video or television programmes protraying a similar incident? Has the child combined a real, experienced event with one vicariously experienced to create different levels of language use?

A crucial further consideration when the child is communicating through play, rather than making direct verbal statements, however, is to what extent the child is fantasising the event enacted simply because it is *play*. Play by its very nature has an '*as if*' quality attached to it. It is essential in making a judgement on whether in his play production the child is basing the enactment on real-life events rather than fantasy, that the therapist is both well acquainted with the child development literature, and the play and abuse literature in particular, and has sufficient direct experience of normal play in children of different ages. It is also important to be familiar with the assessed child's usual play patterns, personality and life history. With this knowledge and experience she will then be able to compare the child's individual play patterns within sessions to those of other children of his age, gender and background as follows.

A child's pretend play with a non-directive therapist can be compared to normal carer–child play communications researched with younger children, in which the carer is highly familiar with the child's usual play scripts and many of the child's past experiences. A carer, in contrast to a child play partner, is well placed to aid the child in elaborating his or her own play scripts in a highly individualised way (Kreye, 1984). The therapist too, like a carer, would be emotionally available to a child such as Ben, helping him to individualise his play scripts, and familiar with his play and history, but in much more general terms. Unlike a carer she would depend upon her professional knowledge and experience of normal child development and play in particular, as well as her knowledge and experience of child abuse to fill in gaps in her detailed knowledge of Ben's life. The therapist would also know that with an older child of Ben's age in British society, his symbolic play would not usually be with adults, but with his peers. When an adult was involved, the adult's role would tend to be either more peripheral, or in the role of a director and educator to a much greater extent. In contrast to these natural situations, the therapist was deliberately adopting a non-directive stance with Ben in order to ensure that his play sequences were not altered by her participation in them. Therefore, Ben was able to enact a more unique, indivualised script of his own choosing than would be the case in normal play interactions. The actions in their script did not evolve jointly; they were unusual in comparison to such normal play in being directed solely by Ben.

The therapist, then, with her non-directive attitude in their sessions and with her knowledge of normal play could state with confidence in her report that Ben's enactment of the play sequence in his last session was self-motivated and highly personalised. It was not induced by the therapist and therefore could not be a 'false memory' implanted in the child by the therapist during their sessions together. It was also unlikely that Ben himself was unable to separate reality from fantasy. There were no signs in his sessions of psychosis or of pathological lying, which may result in the person coming to believe his fabrications, or of any other psychiatric condition. Furthermore, he was beyond the age cognitively and emotionally in which younger children sometimes inadvertently induce stronger feelings in themselves from their own imaginative activities, especially their nightmares and games, believing they may be real.

Given the highly personalised and detailed content portrayed in Ben's last session, it also seemed unlikely to the therapist that Ben had been unduly influenced by vicarious experiences, such as other adults' memories or fantasies, or by video or television viewing. Playing out these vicarious experiences tends to produce qualitative differences in play contents, such as being more disjointed and less 'script-like', more detached emotionally and at times more schematic and verbal, with less precise details.

Children do, of course, often enact plots or 'storylines' from sources outside their direct, personal experience, yet it is unlikely that a child of Ben's age would be able to sustain a complicated storyline, directing his own 'production', without imposing his own variations on the original source. When the therapist does detect vicariously generated features in the child's play material, she then must attempt to relate them to more traditional cultural influences (e.g. fairy tales) or to current media influences on the child via videos, television and films (Sutton-Smith, 1988; Jukes and Goldstein, 1993). She will then have to dissect the child's play contents into those elements which seem attributable to the child's own individual fantasy/reality experiences.

Ben himself did not seem to be highly influenced by other children's play nor others' fantasising when enacting his last play sequence. At times, as Newson (1990) has discussed, children (and adults) can be drawn into shared imaginary scenes with highly charged emotional contents. These shared fantasies, usually based on expressions of deep-seated fears, such as those of abandonment, injury, alienation or others' strangeness, to name a few [and which Bettleheim (1991), for instance, has explored in children's fairy tales] can influence children to the extent that they are unable to separate reality from shared fantasy easily. (This phenomenon affects adults as well; for example, in the mass hysteria of the Salem witch trials historically, or the more recent Strangeways prison riot of 1989 in Britain in which 'eye witnesses' gave false accounts of murders and badly mutilated bodies.) However, with Ben, his play productions progressed from more symbolic figures to a realistic paternal figure. They did not maintain their symbolic content in the last session.

The therapist's opinion was in addition informed by her knowledge that in therapeutic work with troubled children, certain roles and situations can be based on enactments of real-life traumatic events. This type of traumatic re-enactment has long been noted in the psychological literature, beginning with Freud's 'repetition compulsion'. More recent memory research and post-traumatic stress research with children gives added support to this model of mental functioning. Recent memory research points to the likelihood that children and adults represent their experiences internally in a multimodal memory system comprising separate components. One type of memory mode, labelled 'procedural' or 'emotional' memory, seems to be a memory of experiences, which are recorded in interactive patterns, and generally inaccessible to verbal recall (the 'motor schemas' referred to throughout this book). Physiological research, in addition, shows evidence of more primitive neurological processing of fear-induced, 'emotional' memories, which are stored as behavioural and perceptual (visual, auditory, gustatory) events. These more basic memories can run in parellel to cognitions about these events, or 'declarative' memories, which are the type that are accessed verbally (Nadel, 1992; Moore, 1995). This type of memory appears to be fully functional from early infancy onwards, and has been documented in research on the enactments and drawings of traumatised children. These drawings and enactments have been shown to include both consciously accessible as well as consciously 'unremembered' earlier traumatic experiences (Terr, 1988, 1990; Burgess and Hartman, 1993; Hendricks et al., 1993; Moore, 1994b; Ryan, 1995b).

Enactments of these traumatic events behaviourally would then be expected to be both highly spontaneous and highly laden emotionally with negative affect. The therapist assessed whether Ben's play sequence in his last session had the hallmarks of this type of traumatic event. Some of the questions she asked, incorporating questions based on the above analyses and underlying knowledge, were: Is the enactment seamless and without hesitation or is a planned, cognitive process evident? Is the child's perspective of the event the dominant one or is another viewpoint more prevalent? Is the enactment specific and detailed, or sketchy and vague? Is the language appropriate to the event? Does the enactment closely resemble a real-life event sequence which would be an emotionally and/or physically painful one for a child? Has the child repeated these emotions in other play sequences? Do the emotions enacted in the sequence correspond to those expected for a child of this age when involved in this kind of actual event? What level of creative play and fantasising concerning real-life events has the child already demonstrated in his play?

Ben's play sequences fit well with characteristics of an enactment of a traumatic event outlined above. In addition, his emotionally important play sequence was consistent until the end of the sequence with his earlier sessions and with information the therapist derived from other sources, including Ben's verbal statement to his teacher. With another child, however, the therapist may note the child's repetition of an emotionally important play theme or play sequence in their sessions together, yet not have sufficient information either from inside the sessions or from outside sources to account sufficiently for these characteristics as based on a specific real event or person or a fantasy. Even without a non-directive stance, the therapist may feel asking for information would be too intrusive and would risk disrupting the child's play sequence. In other cases the child may be too young, handicapped or traumatised to be capable of providing direct confirmation of these events. In these instances the therapist will find it necessary to look for clues within the sessions and ask for more information from outside the play therapy sessions themselves. The therapist, as explained in more detail above, will also analyse the level of emotional involvement the child has invested in the play enactment. In Ben's case he was immersed in the play sequence and had a total commitment to the action which was unfolding. His intense emotions were then followed by emotional relaxation, which the therapist would expect if this enactment had helped Ben to resolve a traumatic event and been cathartic for him.

Another area the therapist would examine is the extent to which the child's play sequence seemed influenced by his coping defences against anxiety. Again, the therapist would have had several sessions in which to come to a better understanding of the child's individual coping style and ways of expressing his wishes and feelings, as well as her experience and knowledge of normal and abnormal psychology with children. Ben's earlier symbolic play, for example, with the monster and with the puppets, had demonstrated how Ben used both a flight and rescue fantasy, and a fantasy of reciprocal aggression to resolve his strong feelings of fear and pain towards the monster figure. In his last session's play sequence, he again played out feelings of aggression which were reciprocal, this time with the father figure. Indications for the therapist that the final part of Ben's play production was a fantasy rather than a real event were that this part was marked by a noticeable shift in roles and in emotions and by hesitation in Ben's manner. It also became more fantastic and less tied to what would be the expected reaction of the child himself in a real situation. It was also the point in the sequence in which, in real life, the child would have been the most frightened and most helpless, that is, the most traumatised.

Because Ben's last play sequence was based on identifiable, real people, it would be expected, based on knowledge of post-traumatic stress syndrome in children, to arouse more extreme anxiety in Ben, compared to his symbolic play sequences. The final part of the sequence also fits descriptions in the psychological literature of a common cognitive defence which children use to resolve in fantasy a real life traumatic situation in which they experienced overwhelming helplessness. Finally, Ben's play sequence departs at this point from the statements he made to his teacher regarding his experience of being locked in the shed by his father. For these reasons, the therapist was able to state in Ben's case that his play sequence was most probably based on real events until the point in the sequence at which his voice and emotions abruptly changed from extreme anxiety to excitement, leading to highly unusual, 'fantastic' feats of strength and bravery for a boy.

In other children's play sequences, the therapist might not have as clear an indication that the child's enactment at different points in his or her play was due to fantasy or reality. In these latter cases the therapist will have to present her findings more tentatively to the court and correspondingly attentuate the degree of probability she duly reports.

CONCLUSION

Throughout our discussion, we have emphasised that the therapist needs to have knowledge of sound theoretical models and research findings in both normal and abnormal child development, and child therapy. This is required in order to allow her to make varied and 'sceptical' interpretations of information and, at times, allegations of abuse from children in play therapy sessions (personal communication, Dr R. Williams, 1995). We have argued in this book and elsewhere that the non-directive play therapist *in her role as therapist* should already be trained and experienced in differentiating between content and process recording and her own hypothesising throughout sessions, and adept at testing out reality/fantasy hypotheses during the course of her usual therapeutic work with children. For the purposes of court assessments, these skills must become not only more explicit, but also more thorough, in order for her to help, in her role as expert, the court to make valid and informed decisions which will significantly affect the course the child's future life will take.

We have, then, explored in this chapter a range of issues which arise in undertaking therapeutic assessments on children in court proceedings. We are conscious here, even more than elsewhere in the book, that this is not only a highly complex but also a rapidly developing area of practice. We hope nonetheless that the discussions in this and in our earlier chapters will contribute, however imperfectly, to the wider use of non-directive play therapy and to the greater understanding of ways in which it can be helpful in addressing the emotional needs of troubled children.

REFERENCES

Ainsworth, M. (1973) The Development of Mother–Infant Attachment. In Caldwell, B. and Riccuitti, H. (eds) *Review of Child Development Research*, Vol 3. Chicago: University of Chicago Press.

Allen, F. (1979) *Psychotherapy with Children*. London: University of Nebraska Press.

Axline, V. (1946) *Dibs: In Search of Self*. New York: Ballantine Books.

Axline, V. (1947) *Play Therapy*. New York: Ballantine Books.

Ayalon, O. and Flasher, A. (1993) *Chain Reaction: Children and Divorce*. London: Jessica Kingsley.

Bacal, H. and Newman, K. (1990) *Theories of Object Relations: Bridges to Self Psychology*. Columbia: Columbia University Press.

Bahn, C. (1980) Hostage Takers, the Taken and the Context: Discussion. *Annals of the New York Academy of Sciences* 347, 129–136.

Barker, P. (1990) *Clinical Interviews with Children and Adolescents*. New York: W.W. Norton and Co.

Beardsley, W.R. (1991) The Role of Self-understanding in Resilient Individuals: The Development of a Perspective. In Chess, S. and Hertzig, M.E. (eds) *Annual Progress in Child Psychiatry and Child Development*. New York: Bruner Mayel.

Bettelheim, B. (1979) *Surviving and Other Essays*. London: Thames and Hudson.

Bettelheim, B. (1991) *Uses of Enchantment: The Meaning and Importance of Fairytales*. Harmondsworth: Penguin.

Bettelheim, B. and Rosenfeld, A.A. (1993) *The Art of the Obvious: Developing Insight for Psychotherapy and Everyday Life*. London: Thames and Hudson.

Bowlby, J. (1979) *The Making and Breaking of Affectional Bonds*. London: Tavistock Publications.

Bowlby, J. (1982) *Attachment and Loss*, Vol. 3, *Loss, Sadness and Depression*. London: Penguin.

Bretherton, I. (ed.) (1984) *Symbolic Play: The Development of Social Understanding*. London: Academic Press.

Bretherton, I. and Waters, E. (eds) Growing Points of Attachment Theory and Research. *Monographs of the Society for Research in Child Development*, 50 (1–2, Serial No. 209).

Bruner, J. (1983) *Child's Talk: Learning to Use Language*. Oxford: Oxford University Press.

Burgess, A. and Hartman, C. (1993) Children's Drawings. *Child Abuse and Neglect* 17, 161–168.

Campion, J. and Pullinger, K. (1994) *The Piano*. London: Bloomsbury Publishing.
Carroll, J. (1994a) Playtherapy and Anger: A Case of a Nine Year Old Girl. Paper presented at the *2nd Annual Association of Play Therapists Conference*, Brighton, England.
Carroll, J. (1994b) The Protection of Children Exposed to Marital Violence. *Child Abuse Review* 3, 6–14.
Case, C. (1990) Reflections and Shadows: an Exploration of the World of the Rejected Girl. In Case, C. and Dalley, T. (eds) *Working with Children in Art Therapy*, London: Tavistock Routledge.
Casement, P. (1985) *On Learning from the Patient*. London: Tavistock/Routledge.
Cicchetti, D. (1989) How Research on Child Maltreatment Has Informed the Study of Child Development: Perspectives from Developmental Psychopathology. In Cicchetti, D. and Carlson, V. (eds) *Child Maltreatment: Theory and Research on the Causes and Consequences of Child Abuse and Neglect*. Cambridge: Cambridge University Press.
Chethik, M. (1989) *Techniques of Child Therapy: Psychodynamic Strategies*. New York: Guildford Press.
Cockett, M. and Tripp, J. (1994) *The Exeter Family Study: Family Breakdown and its Impact on Children*. Exeter: University of Exeter Press.
Cohen, D. (ed.) (1993) *The Development of Play*. London: Routledge.
Crittenden, P.M. (1985) Maltreated Infants: Vulnerability and resilience. *Journal of Child Psychology and Psychiatry*, 26(1), 85–96.
Dunn, J. (1988) *The Beginnings of Social Understanding*. Oxford: Basil Blackwell.
Dunn, J. and Kendrick, C. (1982) *Siblings*. London: Grant Macintyre.
Dunn, J. and McGuire, S. (1992) Sibling and Peer Relationships in Childhood. *Journal of Child Psychology and Psychiatry* 33, 67–105.
Dwivedi, K.N. (1993) *Group Work with Children and Adolescents: A Handbook*. London: Jessica Kingsley.
Ekman, P., Roper, G. and Hager, J.C. (1980) Deliberate Facial Movement. *Child Development* 51, 886–891.
Erikson, E.H. (1963) *Childhood and Society*. New York: Norton.
Fahlberg, V. (1986) *Children with Severe Attachment Problems*. Dublin Conference, Royal Hospital.
Fahlberg, V. (1988) *Fitting the Pieces Together*. London: BAAF.
Fraiberg, S. (1977) *Insight from the Blind*. London: Souvenir Press.
Frith, U. (1989) *Autism: Explaining the Enigma*. Oxford: Basil Blackwell.
Furness, T. (1991) *Multi-Professional Handbook of Child Sexual Abuse*. London: Routledge.
Gardner, C. (1994) The Expert's Appointment–A Solicitor's View. *The Expert* 1, 10–21.
Gastaut, H. (1976) Conclusions: Computerised Transverse Axial Tomography in Epilepsy. *Epilepsia*, 17, 325–335.
Giffen, H. (1984) The Coordination of Meaning in the Creation of a Shared Make-believe Reality. In Bretherton, I. (ed.) *Symbolic Play: The Development of Social Understanding*. London: Academic Press.
Gil, E. (1991) *The Healing Power of Play: Working with Abused Children*. London: Guildford Press.
Gilligan, C. (1993) *In a Different Voice*. London: Harvard University Press.

Ginott, H (1961) *Group Psychotherapy with Children; the Theory and Practice of Play Therapy.* New York: McGraw-Hill.
Goldstein, J., Freud, A. and Solnit, A. (1973) *Beyond the Best Interests of the Child.* New York: The Free Press.
Glaser, D. (1992) Therapeutic Work with Children. In Wilson, K. (ed.) *Child Protection: Helping or Harming?* Hull: Department of Social Policy/Professional Studies, University of Hull.
Glaser, D. and Frosh, S. (1988) *Child Sexual Abuse.* London: Macmillan Education.
Grocke, M. (1991) Family attitudes towards children's sexuality. In Batty, D. (ed.) *Sexually Abused Children.* London: BAAF.
Guerney, L.F. (1984) Client-centred (Non-directive) Play Therapy. In Schaefer, C. and O'Connor, K. (eds) *Handbook of Play Therapy.* New York: Wiley.
Hague, G (1994) The Links Between Domestic Violence and Child Abuse: An Unrecognized Issue? Paper presented at the *2nd National Congress, BASPCAN,* Bristol, England.
Harris, P.L. (1989) *Children and Emotion.* Oxford: Basil Blackwell.
Healy, J., Malley, J. and Stewart, A. (1990) Children and Their Fathers after Parental Separation. *American Journal of Orthopsychiatry* **60**, 531–543.
Heard, D.H. and Lake, B. (1986) The Attachment Dynamic in Adult Life. *British Journal of Psychiatry* **149**, 430–438.
Hendricks, J.H., Black, D. and Kaplan, T. (1993) *When Father Kills Mother: Guiding Children through Trauma and Grief.* London: Routledge.
Hoare, P. (1987) Children with Epilepsy and their Families. *Journal of Child Psychology* **28**, 651–655.
Home Office (1991) Criminal Justice Act. London: HMSO.
Home Office (1992) Memorandum of Good Practice. London: HMSO.
Hopkins, A. (1984) *Epilepsy: The Facts.* Oxford: Oxford University Press.
Hurley, D.J. and Jaffe, P. (1990) Children's Observations of Violence, II: Clinical Implications for Children's Mental Health Professionals. *Canadian Journal of Psychiatry* **35**, 471–476.
Irwin, E. (1983) The Diagnostic and Therapeutic Use of Pretend Play. In Schaefer, C.E. and O'Connor, K. (eds) *Handbook of Playtherapy.* New York: John Wiley.
Jaffe, P., Wilson, S.K., Wolfe, D. and Zak, L. (1986) Child Witnesses to Violence Between Parents: Critical Issues in Behavioural Social Adjustment. *Journal of Abnormal Child Psychology* **14**, (1) 95–104.
Jakobi, S. and Pratt, D. (1992) Therapy Notes and the Law. *The Psychologist* **5**, 219–221.
James, A. and Wilson, K. (1986) *Couples, Conflict and Change.* London: Tavistock.
Johnston, J. and Campbell, L. (1988) *Impasse of Divorce.* London: Collier Macmillan Publishers.
Jones, D.P.H. (1990) Talking with Children. In Oates, R.K. (ed.) *Understanding and Managing Child Sexual Abuse.* London: Bailliere Tindall.
Jones, D.P.H. and Krugman, R. (1986) Can a Three-year-old Child Bear Witness to her Assault and Attempted Murder? *Journal of Child Abuse and Neglect* **10**, 253–258.
Judd, D. (1993) Life-threatening Illness and Psychic Trauma. Conference

Address, *First Annual Association of Play Therapists Conference*, Brighton, England.
Jukes, J. and Goldstein, J.H. (1993) Preference for Aggressive Toys. *International Play Journal* 1, 81–91.
Kagan, J. (1971) *Change and Continuity in Infancy.* New York: Wiley.
Kaufman, J. and Zigler, E. (1989) The Intergenerational Transmission of Child Abuse. In Cicchetti, D. and Carlson, V. (eds) *Child Maltreatment: Theory and Research on the Causes and Consequences of Child Abuse and Neglect.* Cambridge: Cambridge University Press.
Kelly, J. (1993) Current Research on Children's Postdivorce Adjustment. *Family and Concilation Courts Review* 31, 29–49.
Kohlberg, L. (1976) Moral Stages and Moralization: The Cognitive Developmental Approach. In Lickona, T. (ed.) *Moral Development and Behaviour: Theory, Research and Social Issues.* New York: Holt.
Kreye, M. (1984) Conceptual Organization in the Play of Preschool Children: Effect of Meaning Context and Mother–Child Interaction. In Bretherton, I. (ed.) *Symbolic Play: The Development of Social Understanding*, London: Academic Press.
Kurdek, L., Blisk, D. and Siesky, A.E. Jr. (1981) Correlates of Children's Long-term Adjustment to Their Parents' Divorce. *Developmental Psychology* 17, 565–579.
Lennox, W. and Lennox, M. (1960) *Epilepsy and Related Disorders*, Vols 1 and 2. London: Churchill Livingstone.
Lewis, M., Sullivan, M.W., Stanger, C. and Weiss, M. (1989) Self-development and Self-conscious Emotions. *Child Development* 60, 146–156.
Mahrer, A. and Nadler, W. (1986) Good Moments in Psychotherapy: A Preliminary Review, a List and Some Promising Research Avenues. *Journal of Consulting and Clinical Psychology* 54(1), 10–15.
Main, M. and Hesse, E. (1990) Parents' Unresolved Traumatic Experiences are Related to Infant Disorganized Attachment Status: is Frightened and/or Frightening Parental Behaviour the Linking Mechanism? In Greenberg, M.T., Cicchetti, D. and Cummings, E.M. Attachment in Pre-school Years: Theory, Research and Intervention. Chicago: University of Chicago Press.
Marcia, J. (1966) Development and Validation of Ego Identity Status. *Journal of Personality and Social Psychology* 3, 551–558.
Martin, H. and Beezley, P. (1977) Behavioral Observations of Abused Children. *Developmental Medicine and Neurology* 19, 373–387.
Martin, P. and Rooney, J. (1995) Supplementary (Abuse) Cards for the Family Relations Test. *Child Abuse Review* 4, 32–37.
Marvasti, J. (1989) Play with Sexually Abused Children. In Sgroi, S. (ed.) *Vulnerable Populations.* Massachusetts: Lexington Books.
Maslow, A. (1970) *Motivation and Personality* (2nd edn). New York: Harper and Row.
Mogford-Bevan, K.P. (1994) Play Assessment for Play-based Intervention: A First Step with Young Children with Communication Difficulties. In Hellendoorn, J., van der Kooij, R. and Sutton-Smith, B. (eds) *Play and Intervention.* Albany, NY: State University of New York Press.
Moore, M.S. (1994a) Common Characteristics in the Drawings of Ritually Abused Children and Adults. In Sinason, V. (ed.) *Treating Survivors of Satanist Abuse.* London: Routledge.

Moore, M.S. (1994b) Reflections of Self: The Use of Drawings in Evaluating and Treating Physically Ill Children. In Erskine, A. and Judd, D. (eds) *The Imaginative Body: Psychodynamic Therapy in Health Care*. London: Whurr.

Moore, M.S. (1985) Reflections of Self: The Impact of Trauma in Children's Drawings and Cognitive Development. Presentation, *M.S. Moore Day Workshop*, University of York.

Moustakas, C. (1959) *Psychotherapy with Children: The Living Relationship*. New York: Harper and Row.

Muir, M. (1976) Psychological and Behavioural Characteristics of Abused Children. *Journal of Paediatric Psychiatry* 1, 16–19.

Murray, L. (1989) Winnicott and developmental psychology of infancy. *British Journal of Psychotherapy* 5, 333–348.

Nadel, L. (1992) Multiple Memory Systems: What and Why. *Journal of Cognitive Neuroscience* 4, 179–188.

Newson, J. (1990) Analysis of Children's Statements. Paper presented at *Interviewing Children and Assessment of their Evidence in Abuse Cases Conference*, Nottingham Law School, 2 July.

Newson, J. and Newson, E. (1968) *Four Years Old in an Urban Community*. London: Allen and Unwin.

Newson, J. and Newson, E. (1979) *Toys and Playthings*. London: Allen and Unwin.

Ounsted, C., Oppenheimer, R. and Lindsay, J. (1974) Aspects of Bonding Failure: The Psychopathology and Psychotherapeutic Treatment of Families of Battered Children. *Developmental Medicine and Child Neurology* 16, 447–456.

Piaget, J. (1962) *Play, Dreams and Imitation in Childhood*. New York: Norton.

Pynoos, R. and Eth, S. (1984) The Child as Witness to Homicide. *Journal of Social Issues* 40, 87–108.

Pynoos, R. and Eth, S. (1986) Witness to Violence: The Child Interview. *Journal of the American Academy of Child Psychiatry* 25, 306–319.

Raskin, D.C. and Esplin, P.W. (1991) Assessment of Children's Statements of Sexual Abuse. In Doris, J. (ed.) *The Suggestibility of Children's Recollections: Implications for Eyewitness Testimony*. Washington DC: APA.

Richards, M. and Dyson, M. (1982) *Separation, Divorce and the Development of Children: A Review*. Cambridge: Child Care and Development Group, University of Cambridge.

Rogers, C. (ed.) (1976) *Client-Centred Therapy*. London: Constable.

Ross, A. (1959) *The Practice of Clinical Child Psychology*. New York: Grune and Stratton.

Ryan, V. (1994) Non-directive Play Therapy with Troubled Children in a Statutory Setting: Referral Issues. Paper presented at the *Second Annual Association of Play Therapists Conference*, Brighton, England.

Ryan, V. (1995a) Non-directive Play Therapy with Abused Children and Adolescents. In Wilson, K. and James, A. (eds) *The Child Protection Handbook*. London: Baillière Tindall.

Ryan, V. (1995b) *Reflections of Self: The Impact of Trauma in Children's Drawings and Cognitive Development*. Case presentation at M.S. Moore Day Workshop, University of York.

Ryan, V. and Wilson, K. (1995a) Non-directive Play Therapy as a Means of

Recreating Optimal Infant Socialisation Patterns. *Early Development and Parenting* 4, 29–38.

Ryan, V. and Wilson, K. (1995b) Child Therapy and Evidence in Court Proceedings: Tensions and Some Solutions. *British Journal of Social Work* 25, 157–172.

Ryan, V., Wilson, K. and Fisher, T. (1995) Developing Partnerships in Therapeutic Work with Children. *Journal of Social Work Practice* (in press).

Sachs, O. (1982) *A Leg to Stand On*. London: Picador.

Satir, V. (1967) *Conjoint Family Therapy*. Palo Alto, CA: Science and Behaviour Books.

Schaffer, H.R. (1989) Early Social Development. In Slater, A. and Bremner, G. (eds) *Infant Development*. Hillsdale, NJ: Erlbaum.

Siegelman, E.Y. (1990) *Metaphor and Meaning in Psychotherapy*. London: Guilford Press.

Sinason, V. (1992) *Mental Handicap and the Human Condition: New Approaches*. London: Free Association Books.

Singer, D. (1994) Play as Healing. In Goldstein, J.H. (ed.) *Toys, Play and Child Development*. Cambridge: Cambridge University Press.

Singer, D.L. (1993) *Playing for their Lives: Helping Troubled Children Through Play Therapy*. New York: Free Press.

Spencer, J.R. and Flin, R.H. (1990) *The Evidence of Childen: The Law and the Psychology*. London: Blackstone Press.

Stern, D.N. (1985) *The Interpersonal World of the Infant*. New York: Basic Books.

Strenz, T. (1980) The Stockholm Syndrome. Law Enforcement, Policy and Ego Defenses of the Hostage. *Annals of the New York Academy of Sciences* 347, 137–150.

Sutton-Smith, B. (1988). War Toys and Childhood Aggression. *Play and Culture* 1, 57–69.

Taylor, D. (1971) Psychiatry and Sociology in the Understanding of Epilepsy. In R. Herrington (ed.) *Current Problems in Neuropsychiatry*. Ashford: Hedley Bros.

Taylor, D. (1982) The Components of Sickness: Diseases, Illnesses and Predicaments. In J. Apley and C. Ounsted (eds) *One Child*. London: Heinemann Medical.

Terheyden, C. (1995) *The Sexually Abused Child Victim within the Criminal Justice System: A Comparison between England and Germany*. MSc dissertation, University of Hull.

Terr, L. (1988) What Happens to Early Memories of Trauma? A Study of 20 Children at the Time of Documented Traumatic Events. *Journal of the American Academy of Child and Adolescent Psychiatry* 27, 96–104.

Terr, L. (1990) *Too Scared to Cry: Psychic Trauma In Childhood*. New York: Harper and Row.

Trett, R. (1994) The Meeting of Experts. *The Expert* 1, 35–38.

Tufnell, G. (1995) Points of Law: Recent Guidance from the Courts, Expert Evidence and the Role of the Expert Witness, and Training in Courtroom Skills for Expert Witnesses. *ACPP Review Newsletter* 17 (1), 35–39.

van der Kooij, A. and Hellendoorn, J. (eds) (1986) *Play, Play Therapy and Play Research*. Lisse: Swete and Zeitlinger.

van Fleet, R. (1994) Filial Therapy for Adaptive Children and Parents. In K.J.

O'Conner and C.E. Shaeffer (eds) *Handbook of Play Therapy Volume 2: Advances and Innovations*. Chichester: Wiley.
Vygotsky, L. (1962) *Thought and Language*. Cambridge, MA: MIT Press.
Walker, J., McCarthy, P. and Timms, N. (1994) *Mediation: The Making and Remaking of Co-operative Relationships*. Newcastle: Relate Centre for Family Studies, University of Newcastle.
Wallerstin, J. and Corbin, S. (1989) Daughters of Divorce: Report from a 10 year follow up. *American Journal of Orthopsychiatry* 59, 593–604.
Wallerstein, J. and Kelly, J. (1980) *Surviving the Breakup: How Children and Parents Cope with Divorce*. New York: Basic Books.
Weiss, G. and Hechtman, L. (1986) *Hyperactive Children Grow Up*. London: Guilford Press.
Wellman, H. (1990) *The Child's Theory of Mind*. Cambridge, MA: MIT Press.
West, J. (1992) *Child-Centred Play Therapy*. London: Edward Arnold.
Westcott, H.L., Clifford, B.R. and Davies, G.M. (1991) Children's Credibility on Camera: The Influence of Age and Production Actors. *Children and Society* 5, 254–265.
Wilson, K. (1992) The Place of Child Observation in Social Work Training. *Journal of Social Work Practice* 6 (1), 86–97.
Wilson, K. (1993) Therapy and the Abused Child. *Community Care*, August 5.
Wilson, K. and Ridler, A. (1996) Children and Literature. *British Journal of Social Work* (in press).
Wilson, K. and Ryan, V. (1994a) Working with the Sexually Abused Child: The Use of Non-directive Play Therapy and Family Therapy. *Journal of Social Work Practice* 8, 67–74.
Wilson, K. and Ryan, V. (1994b) Therapeutic Partnerships with Carers and Families. Paper presented at the *Second National BASPCAN Conference*, Bristol, Engand.
Wilson, K., Kendrick, P. and Ryan, V. (1992) *Play Therapy: A Non-directive Approach for Children and Adolescents*. London: Baillière Tindall.
Wolff, S. (1986) Childhood Psychotherapy. In Bloch, S. (ed.) *An Introduction to the Psychotherapies* (2nd edn). Oxford: Oxford University Press.
Wolff, S. (1989) *Childhood and Human Nature*. London: Routledge.
Zeanah, C.H., Anders, T.F., Seifer, R. and Stern, D.N. (1990) Implications of Research on Infant Development for Psychodynamic Theory and Practice. In Chess, S. and Hertzig, M.E. (eds) *Annual Progress in Child Psychiatry and Child Development*. New York: Bruner/Mazel.

Index

abandonment, fears of, 129–30
abdication of responsibility, foster carers, 31–2
absence of principal carer, Patrick, 50–1
absent parent, difficulty in talking about, 103
abuse
  by foster carers, 31
  ongoing, and contact visits, 33–4
  see also physical abuse; reworking abusive experiences in adolescence, case study Patricia; sexual abuse
abuser–child role play, 90–1
abusive environment, children in and intervention, 33–4
abusive experiences, reworking in adolescence see reworking abusive experience in adolescence, case study Patricia
accommodation, 4
acting skills, therapist's, 88
adaptation, 4
  to abuse, 99
    see also personality traits, of abused
adjustment after divorce, 128, 134
adolescence
  autonomy in, 181–2
  emotional development, case study Patricia, 180–3
  see also reworking abusive experiences in adolescence, case study Patricia
adolescents
  adapting therapy to, 172–8
  gearing playroom for, 173, 174
  play materials for, 173, 175
  understanding of confidentiality, 177
adult
  appearance, emulation, 77

approval, need for and behaviour seeking, 45–6, 50, 73, 76, 142–3
  identity, development 178–83
affect, 4
affectionate responses, inappropriate, Delroy, 142
affective schemas
  and physical abuse, 95–6
  re-integration, 101
age-appropriate
  behaviour, 93–4, 99
  exploratory behaviour, 64
  physical appearance, Patricia, 169
aggression, 96, 97, 98, 130
  Ben, 203, 204
allegations of abuse 140–1, 227
  against therapist, 221
  emerging during therapy, 49, 58–62
alternative therapies, 27–9, 31–2
analysis of traumatic re-enactment, 230–1
anger, 89, 92, 97
  displaced, 86–7, 178
  expression, 93, 114
  in symbolic play, 78–9, 80–1, 89–90, 116
  parental, and divorce, 104–5
  Patricia, 164, 169, 170–1, 178
anxiety, 129
  about future, 92–3
approach
  of book, 6–10
  philosophy of 2–3
approval and permission, behaviour seeking, 45–6, 50, 73, 76, 142–3
articulation of wishes, court report Ben, 205
assessments
  for court see therapeutic assessment for court, case study Ben

assessments (continued)
  and therapeutic work, comparison, 206–26
assimilation 4, 5, 6, 24
  past experiences, 124
  symbolic play, 172, 185–6
attachment, 64, 149
  behaviour, 149–50, 154
  Ben, 204
  dynamic, 119
  figure, Delroy, 138, 148–9, 151–2
  lack of, 14
  need, Delroy, 138, 148–9, 151–2
  and internal mental representations, 5
  and physical abuse, 94
  relationship, 119, 136, 150
  themes in literature, 120
  to foster carer, 93
  to therapist, 30, 219
attention, rivalry for, Susan, 28
attitude
  therapist's to child, 38–9
  to play therapy, foster carer's, 32
audio recordings, 56
autonomy
  in adolescence, 181–2
  and choice, 21–2, 65–6, 83
  development of, 65–6
avoidence, 93
awareness, previously unconscious experiences, 24

baby-bottle, role play with, 48
beginning play therapy, case study Susan, 11–39
  background information, 11–13
  introductory visits, 13–14, 15–16, 33–4, 34–6
  play therapy, 16–19, 36–9
  practice issues, 25–33, 33–4, 34–6, 36–9
  at referral, 25–33
  theoretical issues, 21–25
  theraputic progress, 20–21
behavioural
  clues, communication, 54
  deterioration, foster carer's fear of, 31
  disorders, severe, 26
  memories, 58, 100
  signals of distress, 11–12
Bene-Anthony Family Relations Test, 220–1
Blacky Test, 221
bodily
  experiences, symbolic reworking, 185
  level, abusive experiences worked through on, 161–2, 167–9
  schemas, negative, 96
brain damage, and epilepsy, 153

care
  plan, assessment, 26–7
  proceedings, recording for, 221
carers see foster carers
carry-over, behavioural changes to everyday life, 12–13, 26–7
  Anna, 110, 114, 125, 126
  Ben, 199, 205
  Diane, 77, 94
  Patrick, 53
  Susan, 21, 32
change, aim of therapy, 5–6
child
  attachment to therapist, 30, 219
  choice
    in closing sessions, 52, 107, 108, 111
    in ending therapy, 115, 116, 126–7, 171, 182
  choices in play therapy, 65
  effect of court report on, 207
  role designated by family, 131
  therapist's focus on, 22, 37–9, 65
  trusting relationship with therapist, 22
  view of events, 129
child welfare, state intervention, 3
  see also statutory setting, working with children in
child without support, case study Delroy, 135–58
  background, 136–8
  play therapy, 138–4
  practice issues, 155–7
  theoretical issues 149–55
  therapist's personal issues, 157–8
child–therapist interactions, 65

children
    and divorce, 127–34
    introductory visit to, 13–14
Children Act 1989, 213
choice and autonomy, 23, 65–6, 83
citation of research and theory, 210
closing sessions
    child's choice in, 52, 107, 108, 111
    difficulties, Delroy, 144–5
cognition, 4
cognitive
    development *see* development: cognitive and mental, case study Delroy
    level, effects of physical abuse, 96–7
communication
    in role play, 69, 70, 88
    silent *see* silent communication, case study Anna
    with young children, 54–5
    see also language; non-verbal communication
compliance, 27–8, 200
concealment expressed by silence, 118
concentration, 20, 129
    Delroy, 144, 154
conciliation *see* family conciliation or individual help
concrete to symbolic play, case study Patrick, 40–70
    background, 41–4
    play therapy, 44–54
    practice issues, 54–64
    theoretical issues, 64–70
    therapeutic progress, 53–4
confidence, increasing, 83
confidentiality, 7, 16, 36, 175–6
    adolescents understanding of, 177
    court reports 213, 223–4
    and development of trust, Patricia, 162–7
    limits of, 17, 18, 176–7
    reassurance of child, 17, 18, 45
conflict, separated parents, 133
conflicting emotions
    about mother, 73, 84
    and role-play, 21
    sexual abuse, 184
    towards sibling, 73, 80–1, 86, 92, 100–1
contact
    applications, recording for, 221
    court report Ben, 205
    need for physical, case study Delroy, 138–40
    with non-custodial parent, 132–4
contact visits
    Ben, 191, 200
    non-custodial parent, 132–4
    and ongoing abuse, 34
    Susan, 11–12
contamination of evidence, avoiding, 222
coping strategies
    identification, court reports, 207–8
    play sequence analysis, 231–2
    symbolic play as, 70
    see also avoidance; defences; denial
court, assessment for *see* therapeutic assessment for court, case study Ben
court reports, 93, 207–12
    Ben, 202–6
    confidentiality, 213, 223–4
    Diane, 93
    effect on child, 207
Criminal Justice Act, 1991, 214–15
criminal proceedings, recording for, 221

defences, 92, 120, 124, 124–5
    avoidance, 93
    'defensive seclusion', 152
    denial of negative emotions, 107, 109, 118
    see also coping strategies
delayed reactions, divorce, 133, 134
denial
    expressed by silence, 118
    negative emotions, 107, 109
dependence on mother, 102, 109
desensitisation techniques, 62–3
development, 4
    adult identity, 178–83

development (*continued*)
  cognitive and mental, Delroy, 143–6
  emotionally damaged children, 4–5, 57, 95–6
  essentials for, 67–8
  knowledge of, 57
  normal, 4, 57
    trajectory, restoration, 64–70, 92
  personal schemas, 4–5
  and physical abuse, 95–8
  rapid advances, 67
diary-keeping, carer's, 30, 42
direct questioning, 220
displaced anger, 86–7, 178
dissociation from body parts, Patricia, 186
distinguishing wishes, feelings and fantasies from life events, 226–32
divorce, children and, 127–34
documentation for court assessment, 189–90
drawing
  Anna, 106–7, 111, 115
  Ben, 194–5
dreams, mirroring life events, 110
dressing up, 73, 74, 77, 87

emotional
  conflicts, in adolescence, 179–80
  damage, abuser-child role play, 91
  damage, acting out, 86
  development
    Ben, 204
    Patricia, 180–3
  factors, interrelationship with physical factors, 154–5
  impact of physical abuse, 23–4, 27–8, 94–5
  independence, growing, 112, 125, 126
  and intellectual impairment, epilepsy, 152–5
  neglect, 40
  predictability, therapist, 65,
  responses, Patrick 42–3
  safety, role play, 89–90

emotions
  misinterpretation, Patrick, 46, 61
  therapist's role in linking isolated, 122–3
emotive messages, 2, 117, 119, 121, 168
  and video recordings, 222
ending therapy
  child's choice in, 115, 116, 126–7, 171, 182
  practice issue, 125–7
  preparing child for, 86
  symbolic play as preparation, 70
environment
  current, assessment, 26–7
  language learning, 56, 64, 66
  for play therapy, 64–5
    see also playroom
  security and play therapy, 64–5
  socialisation process, 64
epilepsy
  emotional and intellectual immaturity, 149
  impairment, 152–5
  mother's response, Delroy, 137
  seizures, 152–3
events and role play, 68–9
evidence
  avoiding contamination, 222
  presentation, 211
  suggestion and, 223
experts, court cases, 224–5
expression
  of emotions
    conflicting, role play, 84
    interpretation, pictorial representation, 61
  of hostility, difficulties, 101
eye contact, 65–6, 107

family conciliation (or individual help), 115, 117, 131–2
fantasies, shared, 229–30
fantasy
  distinguishing from reality, 90–1, 226–32
  fulfilment, 91, 205
fear of abandonment, 129–30
fearfulness
  Ben 203, 204

fearfulness (*continued*)
  exceeding normal limits, 211
flat emotional responses, 42–3
focus
  of activity, 23
  on child, 22, 37–9, 65
  lack of parental, 43, 44, 191, 200, 205
foster carers
  abdication of responsibility, 31–2
  absence, Patrick, 50–1
  attachment to, 93
  commitment to therapy, 218–19
  Delroy, 137
  diary-keeping, 30, 42
  feelings for, Patricia, 170–1
  identification with child, 30–1
  role, 27, 29–33
frozen watchfulness, 97
future, anxiety about, 92–3

gestures
  communication, 54
  interpretation, 66
group therapy, 27
guardian *ad litem*, 213–14, 224
  progress meeting with, Ben, 199–200
guilt, 129

home visit, advantages, 35
House–Tree–Person Test, 221
hypervigilance, 42, 97, 129

identification
  carer with child, 30–1
  in childhood, 178–9
  with mother, 129
identity
  development
    in adolescence, 174
    of adult, 178–83
  and race, 156
  sense of, and attachment figure, 150
  and sexual abuse, 183
  see also repairing and creating identity, case study Diane
impulse control, poor, 28, 97
inability to play, 42

incident diaries, 30, 192
independence, assertion, Ben, 197–8
independent assessment, for court report, 214
individual help or family conciliation, divorce 131–2
individualised treatment, need for, 28
information
  on child from foster carers, 30
  depth for court report, 208–10
  and initial attitude to child, 25–6
  to child, 63
  to foster carer on therapeutic methods, 30
inhibition, lack of, Delroy, 144
inner controls, 146
inner speech, development of, 117, 120
integration
  feelings associated with abuse, 59
  past experiences, 174
intellectual functioning, 27–8
  impairment, epilepsy, 152–5
inter-generational abuse, transmission, 86–7, 96, 101
internal locus of control, 28, 98–9, 146
internalised limits on exploratory behaviour, 98–9
interpersonal relationship difficulties, 97, 98, 99
  see also conflicting emotions: concerning sibling
interpretation 22, 24
  child's, of violence between parents, 129
  gestures, 66
  role play, 91–2
  symbolic play, court report, 212
  unclear remarks and behaviour, 56, 61–2, 212
interprofessional consultation, 157–8
introductory meeting
  with child, 43

introductory meeting (*continued*)
  with parents, 15–16, 43–4, 195–6, 200, 217–18
  practice issues, 33–6
  with social worker, Patrick's, 42–3
investigative interviews, 59, 61, 161, 215

key dimensions, therapeutic progress, 92
Kinetic Family Drawing Test, 221

language
  audio recordings, observation of repertoire, 56
  development, young children, 56, 64, 66
  development, in children with handicaps, 117
  learning environment, 64, 66
  observing carer's use with child, 56
  skills, working with young children, 55–8
  and symbolic play, 227–8
  variations, 55
laughter, 68
leading questions, avoiding, 215–16
life events
  distinguishing from wishes, feelings and fantasies, 226–32
life experiences and role play, 69–70
life-story work, 156
limitations of play therapy, 136
limits
  abuser-child role play, 91
  appropriate
    Delroy, 146–8, 155–6
    to adolescents, 182
  child setting own, 86
  in playroom, 18–19, 25, 37, 74, 75, 77, 80, 98–9, 145
  to confidentiality, 17, 18, 176–7
low
  concentration, 28
  impulse control, 28

masturbation, 185
meeting parents, 217–18
  case study Ben, 195–6, 200
  see also introductory meeting: with parents
Memorandum of Good Practice 1992, 214–15
memory
  of abuse, 58–9, 100
  distortion, suggestion and, 59–60
  poor, Delroy, 144
  and traumatic re-enactment, 230
mental development *see* development: cognitive and mental, case study Delroy
mental schemas, 4
  and sexual abuse, 184
  see also personal schemas
messiness, 74, 75, 84, 86, 96
  correlation with naughtiness, 19, 22, 76–7, 83, 98
  distaste for, Patrick, 45, 46–7
  Susan, 17, 18, 20, 32
  therapist's reaction to, 37
metacommunications, 70, 88
misinterpretation of emotion by child, 46, 50, 61
moral development, Delroy, 146
mother
  attachment relationship to, 119
  conflicting emotions, Diane, 73, 84
  identification with, Anna, 129
  response to epilepsy, Delroy, 137
  see also role play: mother–daughter
motor
  effects of physical abuse, 96
  responses, 4
  schemas, effects of sexual abuse, 184
multiple memories, sexual abuse, 58–9

negative feelings
  blocking out, Delroy, 142, 143, 148
  denial, Anna, 107, 109

negative feelings (*continued*)
   exploration, Anna, 126
   towards social services, Patricia, 162–3, 163–4
   see also positive: and negative feelings
negative and oppositional choices, 23
neglect and attachment, 149
non-custodial parent
   contact with, 132–4
   meeting, 104–5
   and therapy, 132
non-directive
   approach, 28
   assessment of child, 189
   underlying assumptions, play therapy, 21–5
non-experts and recorded evidence, 223
non-verbal communication 45–6, 54–5, 66, 68, 117, 121–2
   and child's view of events, 129, 132
   therapist to child, 55, 56, 144
normalising 'moral' responses, abuser–child role play, 90, 91

objectivity for court assessment, 225
oppositional and negative choices, 23
overactive behaviour, 97

parental
   characteristics, recognition during role-play, 34
   visits *see* contact visits
parents
   role in child's life, 36
   therapist's meeting with, 15–16, 34, 43–4, 104–5, 196, 200, 217–18
   violence between *see* violence between parents
partnership, 224
passivity 20, 72, 96, 97, 98, 99, 129, 200
   indicator of abuse, 42

permissiveness, atmosphere in playroom, 34, 76
personal
   histories, foster carers, 30–1
   schemas 4–5, 24–5, 101
   see also mental schemas
personality
   disorders, and epilepsy, 153
   traits of physically abused, 97–8, 99
physical
   abuse, 23–4, 71–2, 94–101
   appearance, 106, 159, 169, 174–5, 190, 196–7
   causes, unusual behaviour, 26
   changes, indicators of internal change, 99
   contact, need for, Delroy, 138–40, 154
   factors, interrelationship with emotional factors, 154–5
   ill-health, need for attachment figure, 150
play
   materials, 173, 175
   for adolescents, 161–2, 173, 175
   for court assessments, 206–7
   patterns, normal and abnormal, 228–9
   sequence, analysis, 231–2
   themes, court report Ben, 204–5
play therapy
   adapting for adolescents, 172–8
   aims, 5–6
   anxiety and fearfulness of, 129
   beginning *see* beginning play therapy, case study Susan
   closing sessions *see* closing sessions
   ending therapy *see* ending therapy
   environment, 64–5
   explanation to child, 14, 43, 73–4, 105–6, 159, 163, 192–3
   limitations, 136
   and non-custodial parent, 132
   and physical abuse, 94–101
   underlying assumptions, 21–5

playroom
  gearing for adolescents, 173, 174
  protecting children in, 19, 22, 51
  security in, 64–5
  setting atmosphere, 34, 76
  setting limits in *see* limits: in playroom
poor concentration *see* concentration
positive
  and negative feelings, 118–19, 127
  self-concept, court report Ben, 203–4
power, 155
  in therapy situation, Patricia, 166
preparation time, therapist's, 38
professionals
  other, and therapist's view of child, 25–6
  'rescue' fantasies, 157
  working with other, 104, 157–8, 224–6
projective tests, 220–1
protecting children in playroom, 19, 22, 51
protective feelings, therapist to child, 19, 22
provocative behaviour, 97
psychiatric disorders and epilepsy, 153
psychological assessment, other methods, 219–21
psychosomatic pain, 76, 77–8, 79, 85, 99

questions
  leading, avoiding, 215–16
  retraumatising child, risk of, 220

race, issues of, 155
  and identity, 156
re-enactment of traumatic experiences, court report Ben, 204
reality, distinguishing from fantasy, 90–1, 226–32
recognition, child's feelings, 35

recommendations, court report, 210–11
  Ben, 205
records
  carer's, 30, 42
  for court assessments, 221–4
  see also video recordings, audio recordings
reflection, child's feelings by therapist, 24–5, 35–6, 56–7
  and preservation of undistorted memory, 59–60
  young children, 58–9
regression, 97, 98, 111–12, 126, 128
relationships
  adjustment after divorce, 134
  child's with adult professionals, 36
  interpersonal, difficulties, 97, 98, 99
  with mother, 73, 119
    see also role-play: mother–daughter
  with peers and significant adults, Patricia, 169–72, 180
  restoration, role play in, 89
  siblings, 28–9, 73, 86–7, 92, 100–1
    see also role-play: brother–sister
  therapist and child, 22
  within foster home, case study Ben, 192
repairing and creating identity, case study Diane, 71–101
  background, 71–2
  discussion
    first phase, 76–7
    second phase, 83–4
    third phase, 86–7
  play therapy, 72–87
  practice issues, 87–94
  theoretical issue, 94–101
representation, sexual abuse, 185
'rescue' fantasies, 157
research and theory, citation for court report, 210

response
  appropriate to sleep
    disturbances, 102–3
  to child, therapist's,5 34–6, 6
  to play therapy, 12–13
    see also carry-over,
      behavioural changes into
      everyday life
retraumatising child, risk of, 220
reworking abusive experiences in
    adolescence, case study
    Patricia, 159–87
  background, 157–61
  play therapy, 161–72
  practice issues, 172–8
  theoretical issues, 178–87
  therapeutic outcome, 171–2
risk of harm, through therapy,
    33–4, 216–17
rivalry for attention, Susan, 28
Rogerian theory, 2–3, 172
role play
  abuser–child, 90–1
  adult–child, 20–1
  brother–sister, 79–80, 82, 84, 85
  child as carer, 48–9, 52
  child as parent, 201–2
  clarification of roles in, 34, 68–9,
    88
  communication in, 69, 70, 88
  conflicting emotions and, 21
  court report, Ben, 204–5, 230–2
  emotional safety, 89–90
  expression of conflicting
    emotions, 84
  interpretation 91–2
  mother–daughter, 78, 81–2, 82–3,
    84
  practice issues, 87–94
  recreation of personal
    experiences, 101
  within non-directive play
    therapy, 87–90
roles, child's designated in family,
    131
routines, 46, 63–4, 65

secrecy and confidentiality, abused
    child, 176
security, therapy environment, 64–5

self-image, 99, 100
  positive, Ben, 203–4
self-worth, 99
separation from attachment figure,
    150
severe behavioural disorders, 26
sexual
  feelings, conflicting, Patricia, 170
  identity, 179
  symbolism, 142
sexual abuse, 40, 42
  allegations emerging during
    therapy, 49, 58–62
  and attachment, 149
  case study Delroy, 140–2
  difficulties with criminal
    proceedings, 160–1
  and identity, 183
  impact of, 183–5, 187
  memory of, 58–9
  see also concrete to symbolic
    play, case study Patrick;
    reworking abusive
    experiences in
    adolescence, case study
    Patricia
sexualised behaviour, 135, 147–8
shared fantasies, 229–30
silent communication, case study
    Anna, 102–34
  background, 102–5
  conclusion, 134–5
  contact with non-custodial
    parent, 132–4
  individual help or family
    conciliation, 131-
  play therapy, 105–17
  practice issues, 117–27
  theoretical issue, 127–31
sleep disturbances, 102–3, 130
smiling, 68
social
  ineptness, 97
  interactions, and symbolic play,
    68
social worker
  anger towards, Patricia, 162–3,
    169
  attachment to, Delroy, 138,
    148–9, 150

social worker (*continued*)
  introductory meeting with, Patrick's, 42–3
  relationship with family, Patricia's, 160
  role, 32, 33
  statement, court report Ben, 190
socialisation process, 64
spatial clues, inability to use, study Delroy, 154
statement validity analysis, 227–8
statutory setting, working with children in, 25–33
strong feelings, expression of, 76, 87
style, report, 208
suggestion
  avoiding, 215–16
  and evidence, 223
  and memory distortion, 59–60
support
  a child without *see* child without support, case study Delroy
  during therapy, 87–8, 104
symbolic play, 5, 24, 67, 68–70
  assimilation through 172, 185–6
  Ben, 194–5, 197, 198–9
  as coping strategy, 70
  dolls house, Anna. 112–13, 122–3
  encouragement of capacity for, 64
  expressing anger, Anna, 116
  growing emotional independence, 112
  identification with mother, Anna, 130–1
  interpretation for court report, 212
  language usage, 227–8
  mirroring life events, 113
  parental characteristics, recognition of, 34
  reworking bodily experiences, 185
  sexual connotations, 141–2
  zoo animals, Anna, 112–13
  see also role play

temporal lobe epilepsy, 137, 152–3
themes in play, Ben, 203–5
theoretical basis, 4–6
therapeutic
  alternatives, 27–9, 62–3, 131–2
  outcome, Delroy, 135
  work and assessments for court, comparison, 206–26
therapeutic assessment for court, case study Ben, 188–233
  background, 188–92
  court report, 202–6
  play therapy, 192–202
  practice issues, 206–26
  theoretical issue, 226–33
therapeutic assessments
  appropriateness and timing, 212–16
  restrictions on, 216–19
therapeutic progress
  Anna's, 114, 115
  Diane's, 93–4
  evaluating, 92–4
  Patrick's, 53–4
  Susan's, 20–1
therapist
  acting skills, 88
  anxiety, 26
  as attachment figure, 30, 219
  communication with young children, 54–5
  court assessments, skills for, 232
  developing relationship with child, 22
  emotional predictability, 65
  focus on child, 22, 37–9
  inexperienced, and silent child, 121–2
  issues to discuss with carers, 32
  personal issues, case study Delroy, 157–8
  reaction to child, 37, 139
  recording as aid to memory, 221–2
  responsiveness to child, 34–6
  role, 2, 60, 120, 122–3, 125, 186–7
  state of mind, 38
  strategies, linguistic variations, 55

therapy materials
  appropriate for adolescents, 173, 175
  expression of experiences, 67–9, 161–2
Three Wishes Test, 221
tidying, 108–9
toilet, association with abuse, Patrick, 42, 49
training and support, foster carers, 31
traumatic memories, reworking in therapy, 123–5, 204–5, 230–1
trust
  and confidentiality, 162–7
  versus mistrust, 180–1

unconscious experiences, making conscious, 23
unresolved issues, 127
  Anna, 127
  case study Patricia, 182
  Diane, 93
  Patricia, 182
unspontaneous emotional responses, 42–3

validity analysis, play communications, 227–8
verbalization, in people with physical and mental handicaps, 117
verbalization and therapy, 123–4
'victim' mentality, 131
video recordings
  as audience, 74, 77
  and emotive messages, 222
  explanation to child, 44–5
  observation, childs linguistic repertoire, 56
violence, 97
violence between parents, 103
  child's interpretation, 129
  effect on child, 62, 114, 118, 130
voice, emotive power of, 120
vulnerability, Delroy, 138–40

waiting time, utilisation, 29
watchfulness, 42, 97, 129
wishes, distinguishing from life events, 226–32
withdrawn behaviour, 97
writing assessments for court, 207–12

young children
  allegations of abuse, 58–62
  and divorce, 128, 134

zoo animals, symbolic play, 112–13